THE
STIMULATI
EXPERIENCE

THE STIMULATI EXPERIENCE

9 Skills for Getting Past Pain,
Setbacks, and Trauma to
Ignite Health and Happiness

JIM CURTIS
Foreword by Gabrielle Bernstein

RODALE.

RODALE *wellness*

Live happy. Be healthy. Get inspired.

Sign up today to get exclusive access to our authors, exclusive bonuses, and the most authoritative, useful, and cutting-edge information on health, wellness, fitness, and living your life to the fullest.

Visit us online at RodaleWellness.com
Join us at RodaleWellness.com/Join

© 2017 by Jim Curtis

All rights reserved. No part of this publication may be reproduced or transmitted in any form or by any means, electronic or mechanical, including photocopying, recording, or any other information storage and retrieval system, without the written permission of the publisher.

Robert Frost, "Stopping by Woods on a Snowy Evening" from *The Poetry of Robert Frost*, edited by Edward Connery Lathem. Copyright 1923, © 1969 by Henry Holt and Company, Inc., renewed 1951, by Robert Frost. Reprinted with the permission of Henry Holt and Company, LLC.

Rodale books may be purchased for business or promotional use for special sales. For information, please email rodalebooks@rodale.com.

Printed in the United States of America

Rodale Inc. makes every effort to use acid-free ∞, recycled paper ♻.

Illustration by Karen Morgenbesser

Photographs: pages xxvii, 3, 12, 171, 173: Jim Curtis; page 34: Alan Lee's Chinese Kung-Fu, Wu-Su Association; page 37: Kadampa Meditation Center NYC; page 46: Melvin Brighton-Miller; page 75: Healing Dimensions ACC; page 90: Timur Civan; page 127: Geraldine Agren; page 157: personal collection of Dr. Rosenfield

Book design by Amy King

Library of Congress Cataloging-in-Publication Data is on file with the publisher.

ISBN-13: 978–1–62336–817–3 hardcover

Distributed to the trade by Macmillan

2 4 6 8 10 9 7 5 3 1

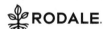

We inspire health, healing, happiness, and love in the world.
Starting with you.

*I dedicate this book to all the
wonderfully terrible obstacles in life,
and all those striving to move forward
in spite of them.*

Contents

Acknowledgments

Writing this book has been the next step in my healing. It has opened something in me—I can feel it in my chest. It has connected me again to emotion and put a larger crack in the wall.

I am so grateful for this opportunity and to all of those who have supported me in the process. Thank you to all the Stimulati who contributed to my life and these pages. Your lessons are invaluable.

To my family: Mom, Dad, Pam, Kevin, Kim, Mike, Jess (my young guru), Jared, Jenna, and Joshua, thank you for being my cheerleaders and my support, and more importantly, thank you for your unwavering love. I love you to the moon.

To my son, Aidan, you are quite simply, the man. This book is for you. And Odie, off the bed—good boy.

I would also like to thank my guide in writing this book, Pam Liflander (you are amazing), my agent Carol Mann, and Adam Mitchell for all of their great advice. And to my partners at Rodale, particularly Marisa Vigilante, thank you for believing in me.

Stopping by Woods on a Snowy Evening

Whose woods these are I think I know.
His house is in the village though;
He will not see me stopping here
To watch his woods fill up with snow.

My little horse must think it queer
To stop without a farmhouse near
Between the woods and frozen lake
The darkest evening of the year.

He gives his harness bells a shake
To ask if there is some mistake.
The only other sound's the sweep
Of easy wind and downy flake.

The woods are lovely, dark and deep,
But I have promises to keep,
And miles to go before I sleep,
And miles to go before I sleep.

–Robert Frost

FOREWORD

I've been a full-time student and teacher of spirituality and personal growth for 12 years. One beautiful benefit of having such a consistent spiritual practice is that I've shifted the way I think about, recognize, and deal with something that often keeps us in a headlock: fear. Now, fear can be pretty straightforward and helpful—for example, it helps to keep us from doing reckless things, like darting into the street. But there's a whole other kind of fear that's very layered and lives deep within our psyche: It's a belief system formed from stories of our past. We've held on to these fearful beliefs for decades, and we project them onto the present and the future.

Recognizing and releasing fear is something I do daily. As a student and teacher of the metaphysical text *A Course in Miracles*, I know that when I catch myself detouring into fear, I can choose again. And I do it every single day. I'm in no way immune to fear! I've talked about my fears in my books, on both my blog and YouTube channel, and even on national TV with Oprah and Dr. Oz.

In the past 12 years, I've learned something really powerful about myself, and I strongly feel that it will resonate with you, too. I believe that on some level, we're addicted to our fears—we don't really want to live without them. I've also learned that if we want to find true freedom and happiness, we have to release our resistance to these fears. Refusing to acknowledge fear only gives it more power. Freedom from fear becomes available to us when we accept that fear is normal, and that we're not weak or weird for feeling it. When you recognize your fears, you can look at them from a place of love.

My friend Jim Curtis calls this more positive, loving relationship with fear "creating vulnerability," and I was thrilled to read about this idea in the beautiful book you're holding in your hands right now. In many ways, Jim and I have traveled the same path. We have both experienced major struggles and overcome despair by finding our authentic selves. The work he has done with his Stimulati (the people and places that have influenced him), which he shares on these pages, reminds me of my relationship with John of God. In fact, it's because of John of God that Jim and I met.

Jim and I share a very dear friend, Jenny. Jenny would talk to me about Jim all the time, and I felt like I was getting to know him, even though we'd never met. Jenny's stories about Jim were always in the context of the wonderful, loving, fearless experiences he would take on in his quest to find his authentic self. Of course, the Universe has a way of bringing together people who need to meet, and it did just that. John of God, an extraordinary and world-renowned spiritual healer, was holding a healing session for hundreds of people at the Omega Center in Rhinebeck, New York. It was incredibly peaceful. Everyone there was dressed in pure white, meeting each other and working in solitude, meditating and feeling his spiritual healing power.

As we wrapped up a meditation session on the first day of the retreat, I saw a man walking toward me on the green. He was moving with a little difficulty, but at the same time, he was glowing beautifully in white. When he came up to me, he said, "We have a mutual friend, Jenny," and right then I knew it was Jim. We experienced John of God together and talked about his ability to bring people together in kindness and health.

I sensed Jim's openness and desire to authentically connect with others. It is truly his purpose. And I realized that we share a mission: to help people discover their authentic selves, to enlighten, and to create more love and kindness in the world. After dealing with traumas in our lives, Jim and I both surrendered our need to control and our desire to escape, and we chose to align with love.

This book is an authentic reflection of Jim's journey. Within these pages, he gets vulnerable and honest, sharing the wisdom he's gained. Trust that you've been led to this book for a reason. No matter what you're facing, whether it's a health challenge or your ability to feel happy, the lessons and exercises in this book will help you look at fear from a place of love and discover your unique purpose. And living a life of purpose is one of the most powerful ways to reclaim your health.

Gabrielle Bernstein

INTRODUCTION

agreed to give it a try. The peripherally inserted central catheter (or PICC line) had to be surgically implanted. A strong tube, a couple of feet long, was inserted through a vein in my arm. It ran up through my bicep and shoulder and stopped at the top of my heart. It delivered a high dosage of seriously strong drugs, drugs you should not be on for a long period of time. Luckily for me, the treatments made a significant difference. I felt better for the first time in years.

Meanwhile, I was still out partying and generally behaving like a maniac until I finally pushed it too far and broke the PICC line in a bar-room brawl. I was in a seedy New York City dive bar when the tube ruptured. As soon as I realized what had happened, my doctor's warnings about the risks and care of the line immediately echoed in my head. Infection. Aneurysm. Death. Responsibility . . .

In the dim light of the dive bar bathroom, I tried to assess the damage, and I realized there was a significant amount of blood in the line and trickling down my forearm. Not knowing what to do, I called my mother, and she said quite matter-of-factly, "Pull it out."

Ever since the onset of my illness, I had worked up a strong aversion to needles and all things that could be inserted into the veins of my body. I looked at myself in the bathroom mirror and thought, "Can I actually do this?" I had a feeling of being outside myself as I pulled out almost 2 feet of tubing. I felt things get dark, and I almost passed out: It didn't slide out easily; there were some tugs along the way. But I did it. You never know what you are capable of until you do something.

That was 21 years ago, but that moment was neither the start nor the end of my story.

Two nights ago, my family celebrated Thanksgiving together at my sister's home in New York City. My parents are now elderly but still, for the most part, with it. My son, almost 9, to our astonishment, ate turkey; my four nieces and nephews, all 18 and older, were like puppies, huddled up talking about their newest love interests. To my disbelief, my sister and I have become the middle-age adults in the room.

This past year has not been easy for my family. We've all had our ups and downs, but what particularly marks this holiday is that my sister's baby, the youngest son, has come back home from over a year of therapeutic schooling in Montana for anxiety and what they call dangerous coping mechanisms. He now has the insight of a guru: He has not only done the work but also accepted his experience and used it to change his story. He is at ease, confident, and calm, and he was the first person to ask me *why* I am writing this book. I have answered the question *so what is the book about?* many times, but *why* was new. I answered him with some bullshit about the power of mindset and how I felt compelled to get the word out. True enough, but my answer stuck with me, because it just didn't feel authentic.

I have been consumed by his question since, and it is not until this moment, sitting in the back of an Uber watching the blur of trees go by, that I get real with why I am writing. The truth is, I am writing this book because I want my suffering to mean something.

I want to believe it was all for a higher purpose.

I know pain . . . well. I have experienced life with the hopelessness that even another oxycodone or Vicodin couldn't fix. I have been intimate with despair and have lived in the darkness of guilt and shame that surrounds illness. I have felt my body crumble under the fight for mental, physical, and spiritual health as my muscles, energy, strength, and self-worth withered away. I understand forgetting what *good* or *normal* feels like. I have been comforted by denial and have made up justifications and told stories built around lies for survival. I have experienced the crush of heartbreak, the loss of close relationships, and the confusion of wondering *who am I?* and *what should I do now?*

For much of my life I let my stories, specifically the ones around my illness and sense of self, define and create my reality. When I finally got clear after practicing the lessons of the Stimulati, I could see what I was creating and chose to create a new story. Then my life changed dramatically for the better.

My Stimulati experiences were the turning points in my life. The skills I learned from integrating the work of the world's leading thought igniters and healers gave me a new mindset that I then made real by the stronger, better, bolder story I chose to live. The mindset is about being bold enough to examine your present reality (caution: this might sting a bit) and not the oftentimes limited stories we tell ourselves and others that are based in fear and inadequacy. Shit, I could have put those two emotions in the first paragraph, because they've been like welcome family members to me. Happily, they are like estranged second cousins now. I became strong enough to accept the truth, which led me to feel better than ever before.

The experiences in this book will teach you to dump your fear. Seriously. Get a No Fear bumper sticker or tattoo if you need a reminder. There is a better way to live, and in these pages I will tell you my own story and the stories of some truly amazing people like you, as well as show you exactly how to do it.

If you are reading this book, you are someone who has had enough and is looking for a change. You might have just received news about your health or the health of a loved one. You may have had a terrible experience where you feel loss or rejection, either from a divorce, a death of someone close, job issues, or another event that has put a cold wet blanket around your shoulders. You may be caring for yourself or someone else. But as you start reading, I ask you to consider this: By your human nature, you are a fighter, even if you are scared, depressed, or anxious. In you, there is a will to live . . . better. I'm here to tell you that a stronger, bolder, happier, and healthier life is not only possible but also just a few choices away.

You may be skeptical that any single book will actually help you. Is this just the same self-help program from another self-proclaimed guru who will tell you how to unleash your unlimited power? Or will it end up focusing on quantum physics and the power to heal yourself with the energy of the universe? Okay, I confess, I believe both: You have the potential to be and do most anything you set your mind to, and quantum physics is too cool to be ignored. However, I am no guru. I am like you. But I have spent the past 20 years studying how to fight illness and optimize mindset.

I understand that the constant physical and emotional feelings of sickness, depression, and pain are real. I don't deny your struggle, and I know that a quick self-help placebo is a short-lived respite. I also know that often, you've made decisions about what you can and cannot do before you are even aware you have made them: Ninety-five percent of our decisions are made in our unconscious mind. I'm here to show you that being amazingly better, doing whatever you want to do, and being more fulfilled in life can be your reality.

You may have heard or read stories of miraculous recoveries or of people who despite their serious, debilitating conditions are able to do the improbable, survive the impossible, and achieve the unachievable.

What makes these people succeed when others can't leave their house? This book sets out to identify the clear catalysts for disruptive, life-altering change.

I have been on a quest to answer this question. I've learned from my work with the world's leading medical and spiritual experts that these people are not outliers; with the right tools, guidance, and awareness, anyone who is struggling with emotional, spiritual, and physical health can have similar outcomes. Today I'm one of these miracle stories, and soon you will be one of them, too. Together, we can disrupt the struggle and the illness mindset.

SO IT GOES

My awareness of what is possible did not come easily. Oh, let me tell you, I am no angel. I have made questionable life choices, to put it lightly.

My journey, like everyone else's, began with my parents. I was a miracle baby, or a mistake, depending on how you frame it. My mother, an emergency room nurse at Massachusetts General Hospital, was told that she couldn't hold a pregnancy after my older sister was born. My parents then decided to adopt and brought my second sister into the family. Six years later, my parents, then in their mid-forties, got pregnant with yours truly.

When I was a child, there was always something frightening to me about my health. My parents told me stories of how as a newborn, I had trouble breathing and was not released from the hospital for some time. Once I was at home, my parents would sit with me each night, one hand on my stomach, praying the worst didn't happen. By the time I was 8 years old, I had a growth in my throat that prohibited me from breathing again, which required surgery to remove. Was this karma? Years later, I was regressed into a past life by Dr. Brian Weiss, the author of *Many Lives, Many Masters*, and appeared on *The Maury Povich Show* (back when Maury wasn't focused on breaking up fights between estranged lovers). Maury and the Good Doc seemed to believe these health issues were from past lives or possibly trauma from my parents' arguments while still in the womb. While this could be true, soon I will show you why it doesn't matter.

Despite these issues, I became confident and strong. I grew up in Brockton, Massachusetts, an urban neighborhood filled with all sorts of characters and access to plenty of no good. To be more specific: guns, drugs, alcohol, and fighting. My saving grace was the pool: I swam competitively through high school, became nationally ranked, and was recruited to swim at the University of New Hampshire.

When I got older, my mother was never one to get nervous or stressed when I got sick or injured, which happened with some regularity. My athletics, schoolwork, and strict father never seemed to get in the way of my attraction to trouble, and I had my fair share of ER visits. I remember a time as a teenager, eager to escape the house, I was thoughtlessly running and smashed my face through the glass storm door. There was blood everywhere. My mom calmly got me into the car, drove me to the hospital, and over the shoulder of the attending physician made it clear how she wanted the stitches, so as to not leave a scar on her baby's pretty face.

During the summer of 1995, amid a period of heroic drinking, drugging, and Grateful Dead shows, my life changed forever. I was 19 and living on Cape Cod for the summer. One afternoon, I awoke to my typical hangover, pulled myself out of bed, and lumbered into the bathroom to shower. As I leaned against the tile wall, the hot water beat down over me. I remained still, waiting for my head to clear. But I noticed something was different. It was my left foot. I raised it closer to the hot water, but still, something was wrong. There was no sensation. I could not feel the heat of the water or the water itself. My stomach dropped. After some attempts to massage and stomp my foot back to life, I did what anyone in survival mode would do: I decided to ignore it. This was my first unconscious wait-and-see health decision. Instead I focused on trying to figure out what had happened the previous night.

I had clocked out of my job as a waiter at a small Greek restaurant around 10 p.m., gotten into my old Toyota Camry hatchback, and proceeded to ingest an eighth of an ounce of *magic mushrooms* before driving to my best friend's house. He was basically living on the beach in a garage, which had become a safe haven for us to drink and smoke without any fear of punishment. As the night drew on, I had a stroke of genius, which included my driving to a local bar.

When we arrived, my fake ID was promptly confiscated after the doorman asked me to spell my fake last name and I answered incorrectly. In my embarrassment and for fear of repercussions I wanted to quickly escape, and in doing so, I crashed my car into the side of the bar as I tried to maneuver out of the crowded parking lot. Then I crashed into another car parked on the opposite side. Finding myself wedged between the bar and a car posed a problem, remedied simply by hitting the gas with no regard for damage—something I was particularly adept at. Then things get a little murkier. I also remember somehow speeding down a dirt road on my old 10-speed Schwinn bicycle. Front tire sank into deep sand. Launched over handlebars, resulting in solid face-plant.

In the process of crashing my bike, I must have pinched a nerve. Or it might have happened during the car accident, or maybe it was something I couldn't remember at all. I reached up, turned off the shower, and grabbed a towel. Hopefully, whatever it was would work itself out during the day. Then I went back to doing what I did best: avoiding.

Yet after a week, the sensation in my foot had not returned, and I was almost certain the numbness was gradually moving upward. When the numbness reached my thigh and I started having migraines, out of fear, I finally told my mother, who immediately got worried. That was the first time I understood that something could be seriously wrong, mostly because my mother was so shaken up. She quickly scheduled an MRI at Cape Cod Hospital, and when the test was over, we learned that I had lesions entwined around my spinal cord. My bicycle gymnastics and wild night had not been the culprits after all.

Soon the symptoms became debilitating, yet the cause remained a mystery. One day I woke up and could not walk at all, like an immediate onset of multiple sclerosis. Every week there was a new issue, a numbness or discomfort somewhere. My parents tried to keep their game face on as best they could, but I knew they were worried. We never talked about what we were all obviously afraid of—that I would become paralyzed or that the progression of whatever was happening would stop my heart. Or, more simply put, that I would die. Every day for years there was a nagging voice in my head saying, *Jim, you're fucked. Tomorrow could be your last day.*

The tension and fear I felt was like living on a tightrope, so to survive my story of waiting to die, I hardened and turned off feeling. At the same time, we looked for a cure. My parents and I traveled all over the country looking for answers. I went for testing at Johns Hopkins School of Medicine, the Cleveland Clinic, the Mayo Clinic, and other leading institutions, trying to find the best doctors who could tell us what was wrong. The search took up so much time and effort that I had to take a medical leave from college. Dealing with my illness became a full-time job.

As time passed and the doctors tried to figure out what was wrong with me, subsequent MRIs would show that the lesions on my spine continued to grow. Was it MS? Maybe Lyme disease? Neither fit the diagnosis, and typical treatments did not work. Each time we tried a new doctor, he would put me on different combinations of drugs. None had a positive effect.

I started to lose function in my right leg, accompanied by more numbness and pain. Every night before bed I prayed that when I woke up the next morning everything would be fixed as quickly as it started. The pain and limp would be gone. But I never got my wish. Days, months, and then years passed, and my undiagnosed condition was labeled simply as chronic. More opinions proved fruitless, and treatments were benign attempts at best. Joint and muscle pain accompanied my lack of mobility and was soon followed by pressure in my chest, neurological complications, dizziness, uncontrolled bladder and bowels, and flulike symptoms for stretches of months at a time. My overall balance was greatly impacted, and I developed a severe limp. I fell deeply into depression and developed a confused sense of self. I was no longer that rough-and-tumble athlete. In fact, there was no certainty as to what I would be capable of or if I would even live. My physical state became a new normal, and I went back to finish college and tried to pretend that nothing had happened. The way my friends looked at and treated me was perhaps harder than administering the IV medication I was sent back with or trying to walk to class. So of course I got a motorcycle, despite not having any experience riding one or the license needed. It was an old, royal blue Kawasaki KZ750. It was uninspected, unregistered, and had old plates and a loud smoky muffler, but this didn't stop me. I started driving, fast. I would park right next to the door of any building I was going to so that I wouldn't need to take one extra step—and have to feel additional emotional or physical pain.

One surgeon wanted to take a sample of the lesion on my spine to better diagnose my condition. But there was a catch: There was a 25 percent chance that I could be paralyzed as a result of the procedure. There was no way that the risk outweighed the rewards in my mind, because once they cut, you don't get it back. So I refused. Instead, we chose less-invasive testing, which meant more spinal taps: not my favorite procedure. They performed so many spinal taps that scar tissue formed in my lower back at the insertion point, causing me even more spasticity and muscle pain.

It took 3 full years to find a combination of drugs that seemed to stabilize my symptoms and slow their development. But I was still left with the limp, numbness, and muscle spasms that persist today. Worse, my self-confidence took a hit as a result of my health. Friends told me that I was becoming cynical, and one by one, they dropped out of my life. To the outside world I maintained a positive frame of mind, but it came as a result of keeping myself in denial about my condition. For a long time, I honestly thought that I was going to wake up and *poof,* my body would be miraculously healed.

I was in survival mode: a state of mind that copes with *what is* and doesn't allow for *what could be* thinking. Before becoming ill, I operated with a cocky confidence in my physical ability, often to the hindrance of clear thought. That's a technical way of saying I was a little bit of, well, an asshole. It didn't matter what type of situation I got myself into, because I could muscle my way through or out of it with relative ease. Well, not anymore. I had to start thinking three steps ahead. I had to plan and navigate the world in a more careful way so I wouldn't stumble and fall. I started limiting my activity. I had to always know if there was seating wherever I was going or estimate how far I would have to limp to a table upon arriving at a restaurant. Were the restrooms difficult to get to? Would I have to deal with a crowd? The embarrassment of tripping and falling down in the dining room of crowded restaurants became a norm. My denial did not allow for me to carry a cane or drink any less.

At the same time, I was feeling extremely vulnerable, so I put up a wall. I wasn't going to tell other people that I didn't feel well or I couldn't control my bowels; those kinds of things were not in my playbook at that time. And because they weren't in my playbook, I stayed ill. To some extent, I went out of my way to make myself worse, because I started self-medicating with drugs and alcohol to avoid reality. I was angry and full of shame, and when people would ask what happened to me, I didn't want to get into it. So I created a story I could

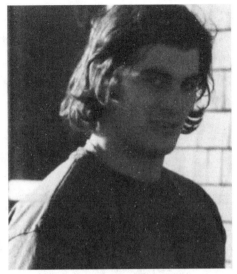

Hours before my family intervention, and days before moving to New York City. My "You Can't Hurt Superman" self.

hide behind. A motorcycle accident was much easier to explain, and I thought it would bring less judgment than an undiagnosed illness. Whenever someone asked, "How are you?" my reply was always, "You can't hurt Superman." In reality, I felt hollow and totally alone.

In late 1996, after a family intervention where my mother cried and begged me to focus on my health so that I could get better and my father lectured me about the risk of the hallucinogenics I was doing, I, under duress, took a leave from school and moved to New York City to live with my oldest sister and her family for a year.

My parents thought that the move would be better for me: NYC was where the best hospitals were, and that's where I would have the best chance to be my healthiest. It was a bold move on their part; they were taking an action in what they thought was my best interest, despite their fear of disrupting my current life, including completing college.

That year, my father sent me a *Boston Globe* article about a woman who had all of my symptoms yet somehow had the perseverance to explore more possibilities. This woman had found a physician, a true healer named Sam Donta, MD, who combined a particular cocktail of drugs and counseling that changed her life. She began to recover in just months.

Reading this woman's story was the first time I actually felt an emotion in over a year. It was hope creeping in. I could feel the burden lift a tiny bit; I could take a breath. Her story gave me the permission to keep searching for answers: Perhaps there was hope for me if I continued to work through this.

I found Dr. Donta, motivated myself to get on his new-patient list, made an appointment, and went to see him. When he told me he could help and that he believed I had Lyme disease, I had such an overwhelming sense of relief. Finally, someone understood me: It was like no feeling I had ever felt. My emotions rushed back in. I almost felt alive again, and for the first time in a long time I began to cry. I mean the gut-wrenching, this-has-to-come-out, am-I-the-one-making-those-sounds crying.

In the end I did not have Lyme disease—or maybe I did, who knows—but this was a turning point. Dr. Donta's ideas were innovative and scary. He told me clearly, "I want to insert a peripherally inserted central catheter, known as a PICC line, into your central nervous system, and you will deliver carefully dosed medications to yourself at home, every day. There's a lot of maintenance. If the wound gets exposed, you could get a blood infection and there is a chance of death. If you get air in the tube, you could develop an aneurysm and die. So this treatment requires a lot of responsibility, something you need to claim. It's going to make you sick at first, and then I think it'll make you better. But there are no guarantees."

Now we are back to where we began: fighting in a bar in NYC, and struggling in a dirty bathroom to pull out my sugically implanted PICC line for fear of catastrophe. Overreaction or not, I remember thinking that this crazy incident was just another day in what had become my normal life. I had no thought that maybe I had to make some lifestyle changes. The party continued.

THE STIMULATI: IGNITING POSSIBILITY

I eventually got a new PICC line (this is another fun story that involves my mother's nursing friend, stolen medical supplies, a kitchen table, Frank Sinatra playing on repeat, and a couple of yapping bichons), and the treatments continued. Dr. Donta's medication protocol reduced my symptoms, and I could operate on a much higher level. I graduated and found myself back in NYC with a job working as a trader at the American Stock Exchange. I started to heal physically but still was in pain, had numbness, was overweight and unhappy, and had a severe limp. However, I now had the drive and curiosity to explore every healing option that came my way, including holistic and alternative medicine. I was open to trying anything that would make me feel better or give me a definitive diagnosis.

STORY BREAK: You may have noticed I rarely talk about how I felt; I explain it, I interpret it. I tell you factually what happened, but there is little authentic emotion in this story. When I read what I've written, it's scary to me because perhaps like you now, I truly could not connect to any emotion during this time. I was so closed, so afraid to feel or accept my circumstance that I can't even remember having any true, authentic emotion or instance to describe.

Can you relate? Just wait, this will change.

New York City is an easy place to find healers, because everybody has one. I decided to say yes to anybody who said, "I've got a guy you should see," and that conversation happened often. My search for answers took me on a wild journey on which I met, worked with, and was inspired by a myriad of traditional and holistic treatments, practices, and mentors, from an Ecuadorian shaman to a kung fu Grand Master and qi gong. I traveled all over the world to see them, and some were right in my own neighborhood. Not all of them were outstanding, but the ones who were changed my life forever. In fact, each one of them impacted me in a different way, opening my consciousness, awareness, and understanding. I call these transformative people, places, experiences, and research the Stimulati—the Latin passive participle of *stimuli*, which means to stimulate.

The Stimulati helped me to realize that there was much more to me than my body being sick and damaged. I didn't know how to deal with this knowledge at first, and I didn't know how to use it, because I was accustomed to moving through life body first: kinesthetically overcoming challenges with my physical self. Now that my body didn't work, I was forced to use my mind. I was starting to see the world beyond myself: I was developing my intuition and perception and, in time, empathy for other people's pain. I learned to be more present and awakened my curiosity into what was truly possible—not only for my life but also for all of our lives.

Each time I worked with a new Stimulati, it was like one door would open and three more would be revealed. The journey led me to more places where I could find more evidence, allowing for more possibilities. I was finding my way and awakening into a new way of thinking. By combining the lessons I learned regarding epigenetics, the mind/body connection, and the power of personal contribution and love, I moved from utter despair, singular thinking, and pain to abundance and excitement. And through this deliberate work, I re-created a life filled with power, success, purpose, and meaning.

Once I discovered my most empowering story and sense of direction and meaning, my health improved, even though there was no additional medical treatment. By the time I was 32, I became an old case that doctors weren't interested in. Yet as I lived with meaning, which I found using the techniques learned from my Stimulati, I was able to increase my sense of self-worth and adequacy, lower my stress and anxiety, and adopt a mindset that was strong and powerful and allowed me to achieve whatever I wanted. The self-destructive behaviors and thoughts that were holding me back came to an end. I learned to be vulnerable and powerful at the same time.

Today, at 41, I'm feeling better than I've been in 20 years. My pain is nearly gone; I work out regularly, including swimming and boxing; and I'm 40 pounds lighter than I was a couple of years ago. Professionally I am a coach and adviser to young entrepreneurs, and I have helped three companies have successful IPOs, allowing me to live in financial abundance. I have fallen in love and have a great relationship with my young son. Although I still walk with a limp and have residual health issues, I now have a life free of *being sick*, limited, and in pain. This is not to say that I never have bad days, but more often than not, I have good ones. And when the bad days come, I can draw on what I have learned to stay positive and grounded.

In 2011, after helping to grow the world's leading Internet health portals WebMD and Everyday Health, I led the Remedy Health Media team to develop and promote patient education and engagement in a different way, going beyond providing flat encyclopedic content. Through thoughtful analysis of patients' actions and motivations, we developed the Live Bold Live Now platform, an inspiration for this book. On Healthcentral.com, visitors are introduced to people who are experiencing similar health conditions yet offer inspiration for living with and overcoming their own challenges. These stories inspire others to discover their purpose in life, achieve their true potential, and then share their own story with others. Our research has shown that the act of taking an active role in defining your story and then sharing it with others is the game changer that can connect anyone to a more hopeful future and allow them to achieve better health.

YOU CAN BE STRONGER, BETTER, BOLDER

The goal for this book is to help anyone faced with trauma, whether it is a chronic medical challenge or any one of life's obstacles, get to a radically better place by using the skills of the Stimulati and recognizing the potential created through the stories you tell. Together we will disrupt your current state of mind; show you the potential you already have to define your life as one with meaning, strength, potential, and gratitude; and rewrite your story.

This may seem like a daunting task, but you are on the right path. I am going to help get you there, first by showing that you already live in a world of possibility. My experience has let me become the disruptive catalyst that inspires positive change.

The Stimulati Experience is a comprehensive program steeped in teachings from the world's health and spiritual leaders, my personal experience and those of others, and science. The powerful tools you will access in this book are based on the latest research from premier institutions, including Princeton Survey Research Associates International (PSRAI) and Johns Hopkins University School of Medicine, and they provide life-changing insights on how anyone can live stronger, better, bolder, happier, and healthier. I know exactly what it takes to change your belief system from *I can't* to *I can*, so that you allow yourself to go beyond what you thought was possible. What's more, by shifting your thinking from limited to limitless, you can begin to let go of guilt, shame, and sadness so that you can achieve joy, awareness, and gratefulness, which turn out to be the most critical components for disrupting chronic illness. You will see that each comes with improved health. That's not only a promise but also a scientific fact. When you change your mind, you change what you create within your body.

A 2013 study published in the *Journal of Health Psychology* shows us that gratefulness brings your nervous system to neutral so you're producing fewer depression- and stress-inducing chemicals. That provides the space for ease, the release of pain, and a clearer head to make better, lasting choices while you pursue your true purpose in life.[1] The Stimulati I have met and worked with have provided me with nine experiences for healing and, more bluntly put, figuring your shit out! These are the tools that will help you overcome the limiting issues that have been holding you back, so that you can start to live pain-free, strong, happy, and with more purpose. It starts with being bold and committing to make a change.

Having a meaning, vision, and purpose in life leads to less instances of illness, but it also allows you to break away from an illness or trauma mindset. That's what I've experienced, and I know that you can, too. In this book, you will learn these nine skills of the Stimulati.

1. **Discovering the Story You Have on Repeat.** Identify your underlying story. You can't know where you're going until you understand where you've been, where you are, and how you got here.

2. **Realizing the Truth.** You are more than your struggle. The truth is, we all have an Everest we need to climb. By living in the present, you

can become bold enough to change your story to one that is limitless instead of limiting.

3. **Reprogramming Your Shame, Anger, and Resentment.** You can't move forward until you resolve your past, including forgiving yourself for your negativity and resentments. But once you do, you'll be able to forgive those who have caused hurt and anger.

4. **Getting from Lovesick to Love.** Living in the present means living a story of romance with yourself and others. Love unlocks the first door that will lead you to happiness and meaning.

5. **Surrounding Yourself with Awesome Stories That Heal and Inspire.** You may already know what you wish for, but I know that even a secret desire for a better future can be scary. Take the plunge to embrace hope and risk by learning from the success of others, which comes easily once you get back into your community.

6. **Manifesting Your Purpose with a New Story and Some Bold Goals.** You do not have to be defined by your current story. By setting goals and meeting them, you can create a whole new story that is powerful, empowering, and possible. Then share your story with the rest of the world and see how it positively affects the way you feel.

7. **Finding the Formula for Healing and Health.** Your purpose will become more apparent when you realize your worthiness and significance. And with purpose and contribution, you can make the greatest strides in enhancing your health.

8. **Living a Meaningful Life.** Living a life of purpose means that you have the ability to create opportunities, and when you come from a place of abundance, you have even more to contribute. With purpose, you can weather the storm of setbacks and new obstacles.

9. **Pushing Fear Aside and Boldly Taking Action.** There is no better time to start to effect change than today.

By adapting the lessons of the Stimulati, my journey, and the journeys of others, you will learn how to find health through stories of meaning, happiness, purpose, and love of life. I know that for every person there is the potential for a transformation to health. Together, we'll disrupt chronic illness, calm anxiety, and create a new story.

CHAPTER 1

DISCOVERING THE STORY YOU HAVE ON REPEAT

THOUGHT IGNITER:

What could you do if you believed in the What-ifs?

Welcome aboard. Full disclosure: This chapter has had many different starts. I struggled with how to begin. At first, this was turning into the frat-boy version of *Eat, Pray, Love,* and I had to reconnect with my own authenticity and real story. In the end, I chose to start with the story of a person who has had one of the biggest impacts on my life, though oddly not until after his death: my grandfather. Poppa was truly a badass. He had a huge personality, and I was enamored and in love with him, as all his grandchildren were. We had heard all of his crazy stories: how he once flew a single-engine prop airplane in a drunken stupor down the main street of his small Connecticut town, how he would go missing for days while on boozy trips to NYC, or how after he returned from serving his country during World War II he would wake up at home, safe in his bed, screaming in terror. We were not allowed to ask for more details about that one. Poppa had lots of stories, but his ability to define what story he was going to live by is what has impacted and impressed me the most.

During the war, Poppa was armed with the Browning Automatic Rifle, the only machine gun in his platoon, which made him a primary target for German soldiers. During the Invasion of Normandy he was shot in the neck and stomach. Somehow he survived and returned home with a Silver Star for valor. Yet all he ever said about this experience was that if he could have, he would have climbed into his own helmet; he was so scared.

When he returned home from the war, Poppa created a new story for himself, and this time, it was one of peace. He made a conscious choice to change his circumstances. Eventually he quit drinking, even though he owned a small-town liquor store. What I remember most was his booming voice. Poppa greeted everyone with a bellowing "Hello, my friend!" that made you feel high with love and acceptance when it was directed at you. Had you met him, you would never have known that he had battled PTSD, attempted suicide playing Russian roulette, or struggled with alcoholism.

Years later, after his children had grown up and moved out, my grandparents sold their small country house (and the attached liquor store) and moved onto a wooden 52-foot Chris-Craft boat. The decision signified another story: At the age of 65, he was changing his life to revolve around freedom and adventure.

In both instances, Poppa created a new story by first identifying what he wanted his life to be and what he could accomplish. He achieved his goals—living addiction-free and retiring early—by reinforcing his story, one day at a time, and sharing as many big, friendly greetings as he could give.

In this chapter, you will begin to identify and become aware of your current stories. Each story is a narrative you tell yourself and others to explain who you think you are on the deepest level.

Often, when we are living with illness and trauma, we get so caught up in our stories that we can't see our way out of a bad situation. Our perception of ourselves and our health creates our reality. The conscious mind believes what we tell it; our actions follow that story line, and

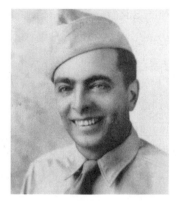

Bernard Patenaude, aka Poppa, shortly before the Battle of Normandy.

those actions make up our lives. Have you ever dwelled on a particular worry and then your fear is realized? For example, if you believe that you are not good enough, strong enough, or smart enough to be financially successful, you tend to leave making money to those you believe are good at it while you make do with less than you desire. You may have created a story in which you're unworthy, a burden to others, or somehow your illness is your fault.

The story I'm most guilty of carrying is that others cannot love me because of the burden of my illness. Walking with a limp and having weakness in my body after living the story of a young, tough athlete left me believing that I was unlovable, and my actions confirmed it. I couldn't keep a relationship; friends and family grew distant. If I didn't love myself, who would? I wasn't really living; I was only living my pain. However, I eventually learned that I could change my story to one that fit my greatest ambitions, including better health.

My own wild journey to overcome illness and become strong, happy, and successful first began when I realized that I no longer wanted to settle. I had to raise my standards. If the woman I mentioned in the introduction that was featured in that *Boston Globe* article with the same symptoms as me could get better, so could I. Right then I began to write a new story without even knowing it. Along the way, I learned that my illness didn't make me an outcast, my understanding of struggle gave me enhanced intuition and empathy, and overcoming significant daily challenges gave me resolve, grounding, and confidence. I wasn't broken, and in fact, I could help others. When this shift to making a greater contribution outside of myself occurred, I not only began to feel better but also found love.

Some stories take a while to rewrite, but others can be created in an instant. When I was just out of college, I took a job as a trader on the floor of the American Stock Exchange. It was my dream job. I had actually bought the opportunity to work at the firm as an intern ticket runner at my niece's charity auction for her school. I was broke, and even though I was paying to work instead of getting paid for it, I saw that purchasing the position was a can't-miss opportunity. It was a tricky job for a guy with a limp, running trade tickets through a crowded trading floor, so when they offered me a PAID full-time job the next fall, it was a proud accomplishment. I told everyone I knew that I wanted it and worked hard to secure it. The problem was that the reality of full-time work as a trader was even more intense than I expected. It wasn't that I couldn't handle the tasks or the mental pressure; the job was simply too physically demanding. Trading required that I stand in a crowd every day, and without exaggeration, I literally had to hold my ground with the other guys on the floor in order to get my job done. Although I had finished my treatments with Dr. Donta, the lesions on my spinal cord were still there, creating weakness and pain, and I walked with a severe limp. I was living alone in NYC in a tiny one-room apartment I could not afford. Manhattan is a walking town—people measure their travel in blocks instead of miles—and it's difficult to get around when you have a disability: Taxis are expensive and riding the subway requires dozens of steep steps to get belowground. This left one option that I considered a depressing haven for the disabled, downtrodden, and old: the bus.

One night, after a hard day at work, I was aching with self-pity. I was slowly walking to a bus stop when it started to rain. I became angry and annoyed. I stood without an umbrella, and I chastised myself, thinking, *I'm never going to make it in this city. Life here is too hard for a guy like me. I'd be so much better off if I moved to an easier town, where money didn't matter and women's standards for men weren't so high, a place where I didn't have to have potential. I should give up and move to a place where I can drive a compact car to a safe desk job and not have to wait for the damn bus in the cold rain.*

And then in my loathing, I witnessed the most beautiful, fleeting moment. While I was standing at the bus stop, a man and woman came rolling by, literally. The couple was on roller skates. Not rollerblades but the old-school skates we used to wear at the roller rink. Their grace was astonishing as they traveled quickly down the middle of the street, entwined in each other's arms as they skated what seemed like the tango. Twirling, water whipping from their bodies, they passed right in front of me and were quickly gone. They saw the rain from a different perspective, one of opportunity and romance, and in that one instant they showed me that anything is possible, especially in New York City. I suddenly became grateful for waiting in the rain for the damn bus, because if I had been in a taxi or on the subway, I would have missed this beauty entirely.

A LIMITING STORY AFFECTS YOUR HEALTH

When your story revolves around negative, limiting thoughts—like mine did—and you repeat it in your head every day, it affects your resiliency: your ability to handle stress and overcome adversity. Without resiliency, it's difficult to take care of yourself, go to your doctor's visits, do rehabilitation, and get the care that you need. You don't have the energy or clearheadedness to make good decisions about your health. Instead, you're left fixating on thoughts such as *I'm not good enough; I'm sick and broken, and I will always be this way.* This in turn affects your self-perception. If you perceive yourself as ill, you create self-limiting beliefs that powerfully impact your actions. Your thinking is immediately transformed to *I can't possibly do it because my (fill in the blank) is a limiting factor to my life.*

Joe Dispenza, a renowned theorist and bestselling author of *Breaking the Habit of Being Yourself*, researched the connection between perception and illness. He teaches that every experience you have and every part of your story create a multisensory memory. These memories are linked to emotions. Whether you are harboring anger, frustration, sadness, loneliness, or boredom, these negative feelings reinforce your memories and determine your self-perception. On the biological level, a redundancy of negative feelings and thoughts activates certain pains, which then allow diseases to manifest and break the body down. Bestselling author Eckhart Tolle refers to this manifestation in his book *A New Earth* as the "pain-body," the accumulation of old emotional pain that people carry in their energy field as memory. The pain-body instructs the brain to release chemicals that can either cause or alleviate stress.

The body's response to stress is controlled by the hypothalamus-pituitary-adrenal (HPA) axis. When we are stressed, regardless of the cause, the brain alerts the adrenal glands, which respond by secreting the hormone cortisol. A little bit of cortisol lowers inflammation, the body's protective resource. But when we experience stress for prolonged periods of time, such as when we are ill, the body becomes less sensitive to cortisol, triggering a constant, ongoing inflammatory response, which can aggravate or cause disease. One of the main goals for this book is to teach you ways to lower your stress response and therefore lower inflammation to help you feel better.

Often, when people experience both stress and illness, they create a story that revolves around this never-ending cycle. In fact, stress and illness are intimately linked. Just as your mood affects the way you feel, your illness can affect your mood. Adam Kaplin, MD, PhD, one of my Stimulati, who studies the effects of illness on depression, told me that 50 percent of people with MS will be diagnosed with clinical depression, while having depression doubles your risk of getting MS. In fact, he's found that many autoimmune diseases, including diabetes, rheumatoid arthritis, and other common chronic illnesses are associated with high rates of depression. Other illnesses including alcoholism, drug addiction, hypothyroidism, and brain injury can all cause depression. One reason is that the biology of depression and the immune system are not separate: They are literally wired together. We know this because there is only one biological marker that has been used clinically to detect depression, and that's elevated levels of cortisol. Depression is one of the most chronically stressful experiences you can have, so it's no wonder that it will cause inflammation.

What's more, bestselling author and world-renowned healer Andrew Weil, MD, teaches that certain abnormalities in the brain's structure may explain why some people develop chronic pain while others do not. I interpret this to mean that pain and illness often start in the mind. Think of how post-traumatic stress disorder physically affects many veterans with migraines, back pain, stomach pain, and body aches. We also know that some people with long-lasting or chronic pain have experienced trauma earlier in life, such as childhood emotional or physical abuse. This is now considered another type of PTSD.

However, your story is so much more than your struggle. If you are open to changing your story and removing self-limiting beliefs, you can allow yourself to both release stress and expand your thinking of what is possible. I call this the What-ifs. What if your story didn't have to include struggle at all? What if your story was an amazing one?

The What-ifs are a much more positive mental space and all by themselves can reduce the stress that appears when you are focusing on what you can't do. And as you've just learned, lowering your stress level not only alleviates an anxious mind but also decreases pain and disease. For example, I find that when I'm complaining and focusing on my discomfort and pain, I will physically tense up, as if I'm holding on to my pain. Sometimes the pain may even increase. Yet when I allow myself to let go of those negative thoughts and complaints, my stress will dissipate and the discomfort will eventually change into some other sensation that is more tolerable or vanish entirely. This state of mind releases endorphins, a different set of chemical messengers that help me deal with discomfort.

Many of the people you'll meet in this book face the same illnesses and struggles but experience entirely different outcomes. As you'll learn, these people don't limit themselves with the belief that they can't do something. Instead, they purposefully choose What-ifs that reinvigorate their purpose in life. And by doing so, they choose to live boldly. Consider this: What if instead of hitting snooze when your alarm goes off in the morning you instead, at the sound of the alarm, choose to roll out of bed and loudly declare, *Fuck it, there isn't anything I can't do*, and drop for 10 pushups?

Okay, maybe that's not your declaration. Find something that works for you. This will send a message to your body and brain that it is time to kick in those positive endorphins and get going.

What if as soon as you woke up you took a hot shower instead of staying in the warm sheets? Hot showers produce negative ions, invisible molecules that we inhale from the cleanest environments and produce biochemical reactions that help alleviate depression, relieve stress, and boost energy.

What if you made a deal with your significant other that each day after work you would spend some time together, writing down what you were grateful for that day, instead of having that adult beverage, which is known to contribute to depression?

What if these actions became habits? And what if those small positive habits had the power to change your life?

STIMULATI VIKTOR FRANKL: A MAN WHO SEARCHED FOR MEANING

Viktor Frankl is one of my Stimulati, yet I've never met him. Frankl was a Jewish physician trained in both psychiatry and neurology who practiced in Nazi-occupied Austria. He survived 3 brutal years in various concentration camps, among them Auschwitz. During his internment, Frankl developed a theory as to why some people were able to survive within this harsh environment while many others did not. He believed that the human body can handle almost anything if you can maintain the right mindset. Frankl identified that the men and women who could hold on to hope and could define a greater meaning for their lives were able to overcome the lack of food, the horrific conditions, and the immense workload forced upon them. These survivors could focus every day, even for a moment, on their purpose in life and their future story. Frankl believed that he survived because he was able to stay true to his purpose in life, which, because he was a psychologist, was to discover and study the human mind. Whether he recognized it consciously or not at the time, he continued living a story that was specifically meaningful, as he studied the human mind under the duress of concentration camps.

In 1946, Frankl introduced his theory in his seminal book *Man's Search for Meaning*. His theory of the importance of having a purpose in life became known as logotherapy. Compared to other psychology doctrines that focus on looking at the impact of past events or inward through introspection, logotherapy looks to the future and explains how human nature is motivated by the search for a life purpose.

This search for purpose is different from the pursuit of happiness. A person who chases happiness is concerned only with the present and the instant gratification of needs. If your idea of happiness comes from having lots of money, big houses, or great cars, that's fine, but it will have absolutely no benefit for, or influence on, your health. The reason is that no matter how big your house or car are, they could always be bigger or better. However, a person who pursues a purposeful life is more likely to contemplate a meaningful future and be concerned about the well-being of others. Meaningfulness is more enduring than happiness, which is why it can sustain people through periods of stress and suffering. As Frankl wrote, "Man's main concern is not to gain pleasure or to avoid pain but rather to see a meaning in his life. That is why man is even ready to suffer, on the condition, to be sure, that his suffering has meaning."

There are three dimensions to the Purpose in Life theory.

1. **Believing that life has meaning or purpose.** Creating a new story requires you to recognize that every life has a purpose, and that purpose is to contribute or create a change others can experience. Your story will guide you to discover your purpose. It will help you create a new path forward and allow you to overcome obstacles. You can't believe that your life has meaning or purpose if you have no guidelines.

2. **Upholding a personal value system.** A personal value system is the part of your story that includes gratitude, forgiveness, letting the past go,

living in the moment, finding significance, and any other positive mission that you take on. In the coming chapters, you will learn how to embody a productive personal value system.

3. **Having the motivation and ability to achieve future goals and overcome future challenges.** This is the hard work of living within the context of your purpose. There will be times when you have to force yourself to maintain motivation, but knowing that you are working toward specific goals or purpose will make the effort less of a burden and more of an adventure.

Frankl's theory has profoundly influenced me. At my lowest point, I couldn't believe that I would achieve any type of success, ever. After reading his book, I began to realize that I had to start to believe in myself in order for my life and health to change. That belief became the focus of my new story. Although I didn't always know where my story would take me, I knew that if I opened a door I could explore the path it led to, and invariably, some new insight would follow. I listened to the advice of all the experts I met, whether they were doctors, scientists, or healers, so that I could find out more. Then, as I began to put it all together to help other people, that work became my purpose. It wasn't a grand plan but more of a drive, an understanding that I was compelled to keep opening doors, going through them, and seeing where they lead me. By using the tools I've gleaned from my Stimulati, you will mindfully create a plan that keeps you working toward a new story and your purpose.

STIMULATI ADAM KAPLIN:
HAVING PURPOSE IMPROVES HEALTH

Frankl's Purpose in Life theory has grown into a new area of medical research that focuses on the interactions between mind and body and the powerful ways emotional, mental, social, and spiritual factors can directly affect health. For instance, just as depression creates more instances of illness, Stimulati Dr. Kaplin has taught me that having a purpose in life creates more instances of health. He told me, "People who have identified themselves to have purpose in life are less likely to get dementia. They are less likely to have heart disease and high cholesterol. We're finding people with MS who have identified themselves with a higher purpose in life who have fewer flares and oftentimes get better. It's because the lack of stress, the calmness, and the drive allow you to be in a mental state that creates a healthier environment."

Dr. Kaplin works with Nobel laureates to create technology that allows people to understand themselves and their emotions and, as a result, become healthier. He is the chief psychiatric consultant to the Johns Hopkins Multiple Sclerosis and Transverse Myelitis centers and has a joint appointment as a clinician-researcher in the departments of

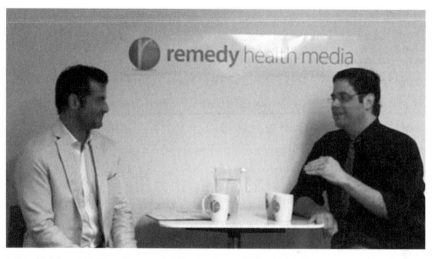

Adam (right) and I talking Purpose in Life at a Remedy Health Media company event.

psychiatry and neurology at Johns Hopkins School of Medicine. I first met Dr. Kaplin through my work at Remedy Health Media. He created Mood 24/7, an application that employs mood-tracking technology, which you'll learn more about later in this chapter. But it wasn't until we started talking about his ongoing research that we realized we were on the same path in terms of achieving better health and quantifying the effects of Frankl's Purpose in Life theory.

Dr. Kaplin was the first to teach me that having a purpose in life is directly correlated with enhanced health outcomes. He believes that it not only helps people overcome challenges but also significantly supports creating the right environment to improve health. Dr. Kaplin has found that when you know your purpose in life, it grounds you and makes you more resilient. That's not to say that all of a sudden your life will be easier or even symptom-free. You will still have stressful days, but you can view them in a different context, focusing less on the episode and more on your life's bigger picture. Knowing your path also allows you to remain emotionally stable and less likely to experience extreme highs and lows. Staying on an even keel lowers the stress response and, as you've learned, reduces cortisol production, which then lowers inflammation.

Science supports his theory. A 2014 study published in the journal *Psychosomatic Medicine* has shown that individuals without a strong purpose in life, according to the PIL test, have increased stress and, therefore, increased inflammation.[1] In another study, from 2013, researchers explored which genes were active in immune cells in people with hedonic or eudaemonic well-being. *Hedonic well-being* means the sum of the positive emotional experiences that an individual has experienced, and *eudaemonic well-being* results from an individual's striving toward meaning and a purpose beyond self-gratification. Immune cells in people with hedonic well-being expressed more pro-inflammatory genes than did those in people with eudaemonic well-being.[2]

Dr. Kaplin believes that those with a strong purpose in life will have better cognitive outcomes, which can increase your ability to take care of yourself, especially as you get older. Researcher Patricia Boyle, PhD, and her colleagues at the Rush Alzheimer's Disease Center suggest that having a purpose in life could protect the brain from dementia. After following more than 900 people at risk for dementia, her team found that those with a strong purpose in life were 2.4 times less likely to develop Alzheimer's disease, even after controlling for demographics, depressive symptoms, personality vulnerabilities, social network size, and number of chronic medical conditions. They were also 1.5 times less likely to develop mild cognitive impairment, a condition characterized by minor cognitive deficits that could progress to Alzheimer's.[3] In a second study, Dr. Boyle found that people who had a strong purpose in life demonstrated better cognitive function, even in the presence of protein accumulation related to Alzheimer's.[4]

Most impressively, the research shows that people who have a strong purpose in life are less likely to die from all causes. One study found that having a strong sense of purpose was associated with a 72 percent lower rate of death from stroke and 44 percent lower rate of death from cardiovascular disease. This relationship held even after researchers controlled for perceived stress.[5] This data tells me that having a purpose in life may be intimately linked to better health outcomes, no matter what you may be suffering from.

Finding your purpose is the critical ingredient to successfully implementing a new story, one that focuses less on your illness and more on your sum total. It thrusts you into a situation where you have to reexamine everything you thought you knew about yourself and all of your priorities. That journey is what this book is all about.

While it's a lot easier to identify your new story when you have a purpose, you might not know what it is yet. The first step then is to find your baseline: your awareness regarding how you feel right now. This includes how you perceive yourself physically and emotionally.

WHAT'S IN YOUR STORY?
THE STIMULATI EXPERIENCE SELF-ASSESSMENTS

Let's start by understanding the pieces of your story that may be creating stress and hijacking your health. While the relationships in our lives are a critical part of our story, the primary relationship we need to evaluate is the one we have with ourselves. The following assessments will help you identify your baseline: how you perceive yourself and why.

Each quiz looks at a different aspect of yourself. The first looks at your past; the second, your present self; and the third, what you think about the future. I hope that you find each of these assessments enlightening. There is no score that you need to tally, but as you answer the questions, you'll gain insight as to how your story may be creating blocks that keep you in chronic illness. For example, if you are living contrary to your personality type (the second assessment), your daily actions will throw you into a stress state, which then feeds inflammation. That inflammation can ultimately lead to chronic illness.

The ACE Test: Assess How Trauma Influences Health[6]

An ACE (Adverse Childhood Experiences) score reflects different types of abuse, neglect, and other hallmarks of a rough childhood that contribute to a negative story and can result in illness. According to the ACE study, the rougher your childhood, the higher your score is likely to be and the higher your risk for later health problems. ACE scores can range from 0, meaning no exposure to child abuse and trauma, to 10, meaning exposure to all 10 categories. Close to one in four people has had three or more of the experiences on the test, and they are far more prevalent among people under age 55. Many people who have high ACE scores don't realize that things that they, or others, thought were normal have affected their health. Many cope with their pain, anxiety, or shame by self-medicating with drugs or alcohol.

However, you can rewrite your story. In an article that first appeared in the *New York Times*, Robert Anda, a coinvestigator of the original ACE study, explained, "In my experience people who have experienced a lot of ACEs don't put it all together for themselves, but once they do, they have an opportunity to understand their own lives better and they can change."[7]

This assessment allows you to acknowledge what may have led you to create your current story and to see how your past might have affected your physical and emotional health. In the following chapters, you will learn how to reframe your story into something more positive.

Answer the following either yes or no:

While you were growing up, during your first 18 years of life:

1. Did a parent or other adult in the household often or very often swear at you, insult you, put you down, or humiliate you? Did someone act in a way that made you afraid that you might be physically hurt?
   Y/N _____

2. Did a parent or other adult in the household often or very often push, grab, slap, or throw something at you? Did someone ever hit you so hard that you had marks or were injured?
   Y/N _____

3. Did an adult person at least 5 years older than you ever touch or fondle you or have you touch their body in a sexual way? Did someone ever attempt or actually have oral, anal, or vaginal intercourse with you?
   Y/N _____

4. Did you often or very often feel that no one in your family loved you or thought you were important or special? Did your family lack the ability to look out for each other, feel close to each other, or support each other?
   Y/N _____

5. Did you often or very often feel that you didn't have enough to eat, had to wear dirty clothes, and had no one to protect you? Were your parents were too drunk or high to take care of you or take you to the doctor if you needed it?
   Y/N _____

6. Were your parents ever separated or divorced?

   Y/N _____

7. Was your mother or stepmother often or very often pushed, grabbed, slapped, or had something thrown at her? Was she sometimes, often, or very often kicked, bitten, hit with a fist, or hit with something hard, or ever repeatedly hit for at least a few minutes or threatened with a gun or knife?

   Y/N _____

8. Did you live with anyone who was a problem drinker or alcoholic or who used street drugs?

   Y/N _____

9. Was a household member depressed or mentally ill, or did a household member attempt suicide?

   Y/N _____

10. Did a household member go to prison?

    Y/N _____

The Stronger, Better, Bolder Personality Test

This personality test is a collection of statements that are meant to help you identify your true personality. Hopefully, it will help you recognize your behaviors and the qualities of your interpersonal relationships. The objective is to understand yourself as you really are. Once you have a better awareness of what makes you tick, you can learn to be more mindful of your responses to people, situations, and emotional triggers. Ultimately understanding yourself will help you choose a bolder, more empowering story.

Get to know where you stand now and you can figure out why you create certain stories. Think of your responses to the statements below with regard to the following descriptions of different personality traits. There is no right or wrong response, and each of these traits exists on a spectrum. For example, you can be a little extroverted or a lot, and both are okay.

- Extroversion is the personality trait of seeking fulfillment from sources outside the self or in the community. Introverts, on the other hand, prefer to be by themselves.

- Agreeableness reflects how much individuals adjust their behavior to suit others. Highly agreeable people are typically polite and like others. The other end of the spectrum occurs when you are more comfortable telling it like it is.

- Conscientiousness is the personality trait of being honest and hardworking. The most conscientious among us follow rules.

- Neuroticism is the personality trait of being emotional. Being neurotic is a particular type of anxiety. Highly neurotic individuals are people who often experience a variety of negative emotions, including envy, jealousy, and guilt. They respond more poorly to stress and are more likely to interpret ordinary situations as threatening and minor frustrations as hopelessly difficult. The less neurotic among us are outgoing and not as judgmental.

- Openness to experience is the personality trait of seeking new experiences and intellectual pursuits. The most open are the daydreamers; the least open tend to see the world in black and white and can't imagine it any other way.

- Optimism is the personality trait in which you hold positive expectancies for the future. On the far end of the spectrum is a pessimist, who tends to hold more negative expectations of the future.

Review the statements below and think about how much they do or do not apply to you.

1. I am the life of the party.

2. I feel little concern for others.

3. I am always prepared.

4. I am easily stressed out.

5. I don't talk a lot.

6. I am interested in people.

7. I leave my belongings around.

8. I am relaxed most of the time.

9. I feel comfortable around people.

10. I insult people.

11. I pay attention to details.

12. I worry about things.

13. I have a vivid imagination.

14. I stay in the background.

15. I sympathize with others' feelings.

16. I make a mess of things.

17. I seldom feel blue.

18. I am not interested in abstract ideas.

19. I start conversations.

20. I am not interested in other people's problems.

21. I get chores done right away.

22. I am easily disturbed.

23. I have little to say.

24. I have a soft heart.

25. I forget to put things back in their proper place.

26. I get upset easily.

27. I talk to many different people at parties.

28. I am not interested in others.

29. I like order.

30. I change my mood a lot.

31. I am quick to understand things.

32. I don't like to draw attention to myself.

33. I take time out for others.

34. I have frequent mood swings.

35. I use difficult words.

36. I don't mind being the center of attention.

37. I feel others' emotions.

38. I follow a schedule.

39. I am easily irritated.

40. I reflect on things.

41. I am quiet around strangers.

42. I make people feel at ease.

43. I am exacting in my work.

44. I often feel blue.

45. I am full of ideas.

Write down a statement that best describes how you perceive your personality based on your responses:

"I _____

_____

_____ "
.

The Purpose in Life Test[8]

The Purpose in Life Test (PIL) measures the degree to which you've found meaning in your life. It was originally designed by James Crumbaugh and Leonard Maholick based on Victor Frankl's logotherapy theory.

For each of the following statements, circle the number that would be most nearly true for you. The numbers extend from one extreme feeling to the opposite. At the end, add up your score. Wherever you land, the goal is to improve your score as you find your purpose and develop a more positive outlook on life.

1. I am usually:

1 2 3 4 5 6 7

Completely bored — Exuberant, enthusiastic

2. Life to me seems:

1 2 3 4 5 6 7

Completely routine — Always exciting

3. In life, I have:

1 2 3 4 5 6 7

No goals or desires — Very clear goals and desires

4. My personal existence is:

1 2 3 4 5 6 7

Meaningless, without purpose — Purposeful and meaningful

5. Every day is:

1 2 3 4 5 6 7

Exactly the same — Constantly new and different

6. If I could choose, I would:

1   2   3   4   5   6   7

Prefer to have never been born   Like nine more lives just like this one

7. After retiring, I would:

1   2   3   4   5   6   7

Loaf around completely   Do exciting things I've always wanted to do

8. In achieving life goals, I've:

1   2   3   4   5   6   7

Made no progress   Progressed to complete fulfillment

9. My life is:

1   2   3   4   5   6   7

Empty, filled with despair   Running over with exciting good things

10. If I should die today, I would feel that my life has been:

1   2   3   4   5   6   7

Completely worthless   Very worthwhile

11. In thinking of my life, I:

1   2   3   4   5   6   7

Often wonder why I exist   Always see a reason for being here

12. As I view the world in relation to my life, the world:

1   2   3   4   5   6   7

Completely confuses me   Fits meaningfully with my life

13. I am a:

1   2   3   4   5   6   7

Very irresponsible person   Very responsible person

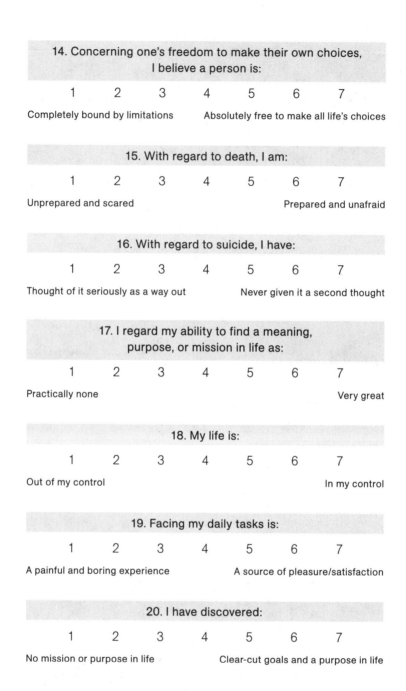

14. Concerning one's freedom to make their own choices, I believe a person is:

1   2   3   4   5   6   7

Completely bound by limitations   Absolutely free to make all life's choices

15. With regard to death, I am:

1   2   3   4   5   6   7

Unprepared and scared   Prepared and unafraid

16. With regard to suicide, I have:

1   2   3   4   5   6   7

Thought of it seriously as a way out   Never given it a second thought

17. I regard my ability to find a meaning, purpose, or mission in life as:

1   2   3   4   5   6   7

Practically none   Very great

18. My life is:

1   2   3   4   5   6   7

Out of my control   In my control

19. Facing my daily tasks is:

1   2   3   4   5   6   7

A painful and boring experience   A source of pleasure/satisfaction

20. I have discovered:

1   2   3   4   5   6   7

No mission or purpose in life   Clear-cut goals and a purpose in life

Reprinted from James C. Crumbaugh and Leonard T. Maholick, "An Experimental Study in Existentialism," *Journal of Clinical Psychology* 20, no. 2 (2006): 200–207, with permission from John Wiley & Sons.

WRITE YOUR CURRENT STORY

Based on these assessments, start to put your story into words. Fill in the following:

- My past may be affecting my health because _____

  _____

  _____

  _____

  _____

  _____

  _____

- I never realized that I am so_____,
  based on the results of my personality quiz. I think it's
  affecting my health because _____

  _____

  _____

  _____

  _____

  _____

- I feel _____ to explore my purpose in
  life, and it might be _____

  _____

  _____

  _____

  _____

  _____

- What if I wasn't afraid to _____

  _____

  _____

  _____

  _____

Craft Your Story with Technology

Technology has made it easy to write your story. Dr. Kaplin believes, as I do, that you can increase your Purpose in Life score as a result of tracking your mood, because you are gaining perspective on your own life. Dr. Kaplin ran a study to see if his theory was correct. He divided the study participants into two subsets: The first group completed the same PIL questionnaire every month but did not hold on to the results. The second group completed the questionnaire every month and held on to it, so they could see their how they were scoring regarding their sense of life purpose. The group that saw their scores was able to reflect on the data in real time and consequently scored higher on the test.

MOOD 24/7

Mood 24/7 is a free application that was developed by Dr. Kaplin in conjunction with Healthcentral.com that helps you track your daily mood and record how you're feeling. After you register, Mood 24/7 will ask you the same question every day at the same time, via mobile text message: *On a scale of 1 to 10, what was your average mood today?* You respond to the text with your number, and the program calculates a graph to help you track your mood, which you then can access on the website. If you miss a message, Mood 24/7 will send you a reminder.

You can print your chart or share it online with friends, family, or a health professional. You can set up an account at www.mood247.com.

Dr. Kaplin's research has shown that logging your mood every day has a positive impact on your overall well-being. In the same way that people who check their blood pressure notice that their levels go down or people who check their blood sugar see better results, the act of consciously checking in with your mood improves your overall outlook.

For example, Tom had signed up for Mood 24/7 at the recommendation of Dr. Kaplin. He was tracking his mood, and within a few weeks he realized that he felt depressed when he was at work. He realized that if he changed the time when he logged his mood, overall, he was less depressed. He experimented and changed the check-in time from noon, when he was at a job he hated, to 6 p.m., when he was home with his fiancée. When the time came to log in, he would consciously say to himself, *I'm going to leave all the baggage from work at the office, and I'm going to enjoy the fact that I have this wonderful life at home.* This small change turned out to be therapeutic, and he was able to log a higher number at home and handle the stresses at work better, knowing that there was something positive for him to look forward to at the end of the day.

What If Your Story Was Bolder?

Now that you are clear on your current story, you can start to think about what you want a new story to look like. The choices are limitless and entirely personal. It could be something as clear as *I want to be pain free and active* or *my depression won't hold me back from having great relationships.* Or it could be something along the lines of the What-if image you hold for yourself, if you were operating at your highest potential for health, wealth, relationships, and happiness.

You already live in a world full of possibility; living your future story starts in your mind. You may not be an executive or CEO, but that doesn't mean you can't start dressing for the role when you're a junior manager. You need to define what you'd like and then start to live boldly now. I wasn't ready to design my future until I realized that I was more than my body. It took me a long time to understand that we are our bodies in conjunction with our minds and our purpose. Today my story is one of strength, kindness, and love. There is nothing I cannot do, no limitation that will stop me, no obstacle I can't overcome. I am a great father, and I can give to others without worrying about loss. What's your story?

To me, living boldly means breaking free from chronic disease, and that starts in your mind. I firmly believe you are only chronically ill if you label yourself so. Even though I've never been so strong, healthy, and in such a great shape in the last 22 years, I still have nerve damage to my spinal cord. I've learned that my physical condition doesn't limit or define what I can do or my hamper my spirit to succeed.

IF KATE CAN FIND PURPOSE, SO CAN YOU!

My friend Kate Milliken started a business called MyCounterpane.com, an online community for people with multiple sclerosis. Kate believes that her MS is under control because she changed her mindset. Here is her story.

At the age of 35, when I was single, I got a monster curve ball: I was diagnosed with MS. Because of my job as a testimonial video producer, I understood intrinsically the huge power of showcasing a story in video. So when I was diagnosed, I went online and figured out what MS was in less than an hour. But I was really looking for one moment in somebody's true life experience, captured on video, that could give me a sense of perspective. I wanted to see somebody who was living with MS, going through what I could expect to experience, and show me that my life was going to stabilize and actually be awesome. But I couldn't find it. I felt isolated and alone. My life was not going to work out.

When I was diagnosed with MS, I had fatigue and numbness, but the scariest part of my symptoms was the delay on my left side. Even though my brain was saying, *Right, left, right, left*, my left side wasn't tracking properly. By the time I got to the neurologist, I couldn't keep my balance. This all happened in a period of 6 days, which is fairly unusual for MS.

Soon after, I met an incredible osteopath who couldn't give two shits that I had MS. He was like, "Why do you have it? MS is an inflammation of the central nervous system. What might be inflaming you?" Even in that moment. If you're going to talk about breaking a mindset, I can give you numerous examples of *wow, you just reframed MS in an interesting way.*

My osteopath doesn't use the word *disease.* He said, "Your body's going through an interesting process." These are subtleties that in my time of vulnerability I grabbed onto. He found through his own testing that I had high levels of mercury in my system, and I had bad bacteria in my gut. I wasn't processing nutrients appropriately. He told me that if he could remove the mercury and bad bacteria, I would heal myself.

He also said, "You know, for what it's worth, I have gone to med school and I have learned that you cannot reverse myelin damage, but I've seen it happen in my practice and I would plan on it." The moment he said that, I thought, *Another moment of breaking the mindset.* It changed my perspective from sickness into health. I ended up taking supplements as well as following a conventional medicine protocol. I also treated myself well, took naps, ate better, and started living in the present. I was so convinced that I was going to reverse the lesion that I brought a camera crew into the hospital for my first-year MRI follow-up. They thought I was nuts. I went in and they pulled out the MRI, and there was nothing there.

Because I'm a testimonial video producer, I ended up putting my own story on a website called Katescounterpane.com. There are 32 mini films that total 40 minutes of time. I literally threw it out to maybe 50 people in my life, and I said, "I put this out because I needed to do it." I didn't even put it on YouTube until 2 years ago. Since then, I've had 55,000 unique visitors, and 65 percent of them watched all 40 minutes of my story. If that isn't a sign that other people need to tell their stories the way I did, I don't know what is. So I went on Indiegogo and I raised $60,000 in 50 days, and then I launched MyCounterpane. Mycounterpane.com caters to three different communities: people with MS, people with mental health issues, and veterans, which is new. We are also launching a community for parents of terminally ill children. I would love nothing more than to have a community for every chronic illness. When we rebuild, one of the things we're going to be able to do is turn on a community at the click of a button.

Today I'm married to an incredible guy, living in a beautiful place with two young kids, and pursuing my dream. My husband married me because he loved me for me. The MS didn't factor into his life or our life together.

THOUGHT IGNITER

If one lights a fire for others, it will also brighten one's own way.

—NICHIREN, 13TH-CENTURY BUDDHIST SAGE

CHAPTER 2

REALIZING THE TRUTH

THOUGHT IGNITER:

Time is precious, but truth is more precious than time.

–Benjamin Disraeli

A recurring Stimulati lesson taught me that your story is what you think and feel; it is the manifestation of your beliefs and what you believe to be your truth, and it's the basis for your perception of reality. Say, for example, one of your stories is that you were in a car accident and now you are too injured or disabled to be physically active. Then you will remain focused on all the things you can't do, and your truth will be your limits. If your story is *I'm overweight because I'm too busy to exercise*, worthlessness becomes your truth, and consequently, your weight will be your reality. The more times you repeat your story, the more powerful it becomes, and as with any habit, it's now ingrained in your thinking. However, you don't have to be the poor disabled guy who can't participate or the fat lady. You can be the guy who is tough enough to train for the Paralympics despite his injury or the sexy vixen who is confident enough to wear any dress she wants.

Test this out. Listen to the recurring themes of stories people tell in your life. How do they then translate to their relationships, work, and health?

Recognizing that you already have a story and then changing it takes courage and is the first step in healing. The goals for this chapter are:

1. To accept and be aware of what is true and real

2. To recognize and then recast the negative voice in your head that is likely keeping you in a place of saying, *I can't*

3. To quiet that voice and replace it with a new narrative that is aligned with the universal truths

The first truth is: You can, and do, control your future and your current reality based on your beliefs, no matter how you feel physically or emotionally. You can rewrite your story and create one that allows you to live bolder and dramatically change your health. A story full of opportunity and ease is one in which the truth is not limiting but limitless.

IS YOUR STORY STUCK IN SURVIVAL MODE?

During the first few years of my illness, I lived in denial. I sincerely believed that I would wake up one morning and be completely fine. I would respond to queries about my health with a flippant, "You can't hurt Superman." Denial can take the form of what I call survival mode, a powerful coping mechanism that lets you get through the earliest and most painful or upsetting stages of illness or trauma. Survival mode is an acceptance of your current circumstance, and denial of what could happen. It helps anyone who is traumatized, whether they are newly diagnosed, soldiers traumatized by war, or parents faced with the loss of a child. Consider whether you are in survival mode if you have become okay with your current state of being, even though you don't have awareness of what is or what can be.

Healing starts once you break out of survival mode. Problem numero uno is that we get stuck living in survival mode far longer than we should. When I was in survival mode, I accepted as fact that my illness was chronic and I would be sick forever. I stopped doing the things my doctors told me would help me to get better, such as physical therapy. Instead, when a new symptom would arise, I would create a new story around that symptom, and then accept where I was without looking for a way out. This was particularly effective when I was in pain. I used to say pain is relative, meaning that everyone has a threshold which that they can tolerate. When I developed lower back pain that led to stiffness in my legs, I accepted it as something that was caused by my limp, and I learned to live with it without doing anything about it.

However, the truth is that pain is not relative. That's survival mode talking, and once I was able to get out of it, I called bullshit on myself. Pain affects our muscles and reflexes automatically, just like breathing. The body instinctively tries to fight pain and heal wounds through the process of inflammation. When you're in pain, your body is fighting a symptom—no matter how much you think you can handle it.

When I accepted this fact, that I was in pain, and that there was probably something I could do about it, I started chiropractic and acupuncture treatments along with developing a regular stretching routine at home. And guess what? Once I started taking care of myself and addressing the pain, it went away to such an extent that for the first time I could not only bend over and pick things up—something I would have never dared to try—I also began to weight train. And with that, I regained an emotional and a physical sense of power and control.

Had I let go of survival mode earlier, I would have healed much quicker more quickly, because I would have taken care of myself. I would have gone to the doctor when I was in pain or when new symptoms occurred, and I would have listened to his or her advice. I would have tried physical therapy much sooner. I would have been refitted for a new leg brace instead of keeping one for 10 years, even as my body and my symptoms continued to change.

STIMULATI ALAN LEE: THERE IS MORE TO HEALING THAN MEETS THE EYE

I met Alan Lee, a grand master of kung fu, at the beginning of my journey. He taught me about healing energy, karma, and discipline. At the time, he looked ageless but must have been at least 60 years old, having come to America in 1959. He is still teaching today. One of his lesser legends is that he once took a road trip with some of his students to a spiritual retreat, and he didn't stir in his seat at all during the 7-hour drive. He was so poised and powerful and calm that he didn't need to.

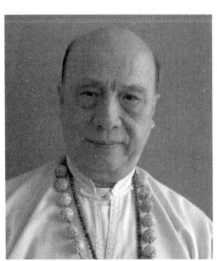
One of my first Stimulati, Grand Master Alan Lee.

I got to know him when he started doing energy work and Dao Yin Bi Ji with me. I would visit him in his studio in Chinatown once a week. He would put his hands on my head and explain that he was sending lightning bolts of Qi (energy) through my chakras to try to clear out disease or old karma. Then he'd tell me to rate my pain on a scale of 1 to 10. He'd say, "When it gets to a 10 in painfulness you tell me, and I'll stop."

Grand Master would put me in a meditative state as he was doing his energy work, and he suggested that I create my own meditation practice. At first I didn't expect to feel anything, but I can tell you for a fact that I felt a jolt of electricity going through my body and real pain while he was working on me. When he stopped, all I could feel was ease. During the treatment I would see lights and color, and old memories would come up that he'd say he was bringing up and removing. It helped me realize that there was more that was keeping me unwell beyond my body. He suggested I had blocks from past lives.

To be honest, I'm not sure it had a huge impact on my recovery. However, it opened my mind to finding the next avenue to a possible cure. I believe he removed emotional blocks that were holding me back, spiritually and mentally. From there I went on to find great opportunities that would allow me to physically heal, opportunities that I wouldn't have even looked for without this experience.

STIMULATI KADAM MORTEN CLAUSEN: A QUICK LOOK INTO BUDDHISM'S TRUTHS

Buddhism teaches that there are two important truths, and I was taught them a number of years ago when I was on a Buddhist retreat. I had already been working with Lee and had started meditating on my own when my friends invited me to join a small Buddhist mediation class in the East Village. I learned an amazing meditation called the *Metta Bhavana*, which is meant to cultivate loving-kindness (I've included it on page 41). This meditation had such a profound effect on me that it opened a door for me on my journey toward healing. My friends and I started going to the Kadampa Meditation Center in New York City, a larger, more established Buddhist center, which is where I met Kadam Morten Clausen.

Kadam Morten Clausen is a leader of the New Kadampa Tradition and a resident teacher at the Kadampa Meditation Center. He became one of my Stimulati through the classes I took with him. Kadam Morten's teaching style made the Buddha's insights accessible. Many of us thought that he must have been a stand-up comic in a past life, or at least a past profession.

In this temple, there are typically more than 100 people following his guided meditations and learning Buddhist principles. It's an incredibly empowering feeling to be meditating with so many people. The act of being surrounded by people doing the same thing at the same time always made me feel connected and less alone.

Kadam Morten taught me the first universal truth, which is that we are all suffering. Every one of us has struggles and burdens, anxieties and concerns. We all have heartaches or real aches and pains. And while it may seem that your suffering is the most burdensome, no single person's suffering is more or less than someone else's. You may know someone dying of cancer or see someone in pain; meanwhile I'm walking with a limp. While I'm not dying, I might believe that I'm suffering more, because it's hard to be empathetic when you're in survival mode. While it is safe to say that some obstacles are bigger than others (dealing with cancer is a larger obstacle than paying the water bill), simply put: We all got the same shit.

Knowing that other people were suffering allowed me to feel that we are all somehow connected in this suffering. This knowledge gave me permission to express a fuller range of emotions. Over time, I started to develop a greater sense of empathy, which then shifted me out of survival mode. Instead of wanting to be alone, I became more connected to others. Healing became easier when I had a community that I could relate to and be inspired by.

I also learned that there is an underlying purpose in our collective suffering: It helps us grow and learn. The way that we think about even everyday obstacles changes the way we think about ourselves and the way we live our lives. As we succeed, we gain courage and knowledge and become empowered, happy, loving, and grateful. Your suffering is exactly what can change the story of your pain to one of purpose and strength.

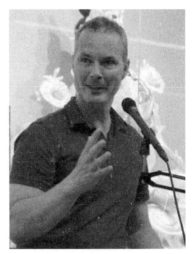

Kadam Morten teaching, in his unique humor-infused way, at the Kadampa Meditation Center in New York City.

What's more, suffering doesn't have to carry a stigma. If everyone is suffering, you haven't been singled out as someone who is wrong or bad, lazy or stupid. You haven't been punished by a higher power. We're all in this together. Instead of saying *why me?* you can free your mind to see the possibilities that are waiting for you.

The Second Truth: The Only Time That Exists Is Now

As I began to fully understand this truth, I questioned the underlying intention: *If everyone is suffering, why are there plenty of people with happy and fulfilled lives? Why doesn't everyone feel like I do: depressed and anxious? How can these states exist at the same time? How can we all be struggling, yet some people are at ease?*

The simple answer is that even though we're all suffering, we can redefine our story by learning the second truth, which is the idea that the only time that exists is now. When I understood this truth, I began to see that the people in my life I considered to be the happiest were the ones who could live in the present. They make choices that are separate from both their past and their future, and because of this one mindset switch, their suffering doesn't hold them back or affect them as much.

The past is gone, and it will never return: Whatever happened that caused your pain or illness is an event that is no longer occurring. The future hasn't happened yet, so you can't know how you are going to feel a minute from now, a day from now, or even a year from now. So if the past is over and the future doesn't exist, the only time that is important is right now.

The truth that the past—the cause of your current situation—no longer matters is not easy to hear. If you were in a terrible car accident, you might be thinking, *Screw you, Jim. That accident really happened, and I'm in real pain.*

I'm not suggesting in any way that your pain doesn't exist, your condition doesn't exist, or that there wasn't a real catalyst that caused you to be in the place you're at. But I am saying that the accident happened in the past, and the wreckage has been cleaned up. You can't go back and see that accident. The only place it exists is in your story. With this awareness, you can start to release that accident from your anxieties,

---

STORY BREAK: Challenges and obstacles are meant to be overcome. They are what make us stronger, better, and bolder. Consider changing the story of your suffering, trauma, or illness. What if these are all tests for us to overcome so we learn what gives us meaning and purpose in life? When we exercise, we first tear down our muscles so they can then grow larger and stronger.

---

accept that it happened, and then create a new story that will fit your new reality. If you can't release your past story of pain and suffering, then you are literally placing your past into the now, and you'll never create a new story that reflects what your present can and should be.

If the future doesn't yet exist, there's little point in worrying about it. If you are doing the right things that are aligned with your new story, including taking the best care of yourself, the future will be okay. That doesn't mean you can't plan for the future, but you need to implement that plan in the present. As a good friend of mine says, "Hope is not a success strategy." You can always hope that good things are going to happen for you, but you need to do the work to make those dreams come true.

Living in the now gives us permission to think boldly about our future, to understand that if the truth is based on the perception of our story, then we can flip the model and change our story to work within the context of the truth. For instance, we all feel anxious at times, worrying about something that hasn't happened yet. Whether we are waiting for test results or even a text message, our story becomes one of us thinking, *I'm not good enough*. We come up with a million reasons, and we're overwhelmed with negative thoughts about ourselves, such as *she doesn't like me enough to text*; *I'm not lovable*; *she's with someone else*. Yet in your present moment, none of those thoughts can be true. That's why if you focus on the now, it doesn't matter why someone hasn't texted you back.

When you live in the present, every second provides the opportunity to define how you want to live. You are constantly living in the now. However, the truth stays the same. I learned that it takes work every day to stay true to my present story. Whenever I'm feeling anxious, I remind myself of my current story: I'm calm and confident, and everything is going to work out well for me. I understand that I'm not the only one suffering and that I can't be worried about something that hasn't happened yet. I have a choice in how I can live; I can make now whatever I want it to be, and when I do, my story can change.

LENE ANDERSEN GRATEFULLY FINDS BEAUTY EVERYWHERE

Kadam Morten's truth teachings are best exemplified by Lene Andersen, a wonderful woman I met when we created a documentary about her life at Healthcentral.com. Lene was diagnosed with rheumatoid arthritis (RA) when she was just 10 years old, and because she was in so much pain and was so fragile, her doctor decided that the best course of action was to put her in a full-body cast. Unfortunately, instead of protecting her, the cast created an environment in which every joint in her body fused together. When the cast was removed, Lene was paralyzed: She couldn't walk, and she's never regained her mobility.

Lene's story could easily be one of disappointment and despair. Yet her story is not *I'm in pain, and I'm in a wheelchair; I can't do this.*

Most days, Lene wakes up, gets into her electric wheelchair, and explores her Toronto neighborhood. Her wheelchair takes her wherever she needs to go, although she admits the ride is often uncomfortable. On her daily journey, she challenges herself to find something of beauty to photograph: a tree, bird, sunset, or leaf. Within that beauty she feels gratitude, and even though she is suffering, her gratitude allows her to be happy and healthy.

A few years ago, Lene started taking biologic medication that better treats her RA symptoms. I believe that the combination of the new medication and her positive attitude allowed her to release much of her pain and even regain some movement. She still recognizes that every day is an obstacle and that she will always have obstacles to overcome, but she is not living in the suffering mindset. She is never going to get out of her wheelchair, but she is expanding the physical space that she can explore. What's more, she doesn't consider herself to be chronically ill, because she doesn't have the chronically ill story of limitations and *I can't, I'm not* thinking.

Lene's story changed again when she began connecting with others in the RA community. Even before we met, she was already well-known in RA support groups and chats on the Internet. She started blogging on the Health Central community forum for RA, providing both advice and inspiration. Today she has hundreds of thousands of people who read her blog and find her message uplifting. People trust her. They see that if she can be a productive member of society, then so can they. Sharing her story has given her a tremendous purpose.

In short, Lene has changed her story and accepted the truth of living completely in the present. By doing so, she has been able to change the perspective of many other people suffering from the same disease. Her photography is poignant, but her purpose has become to tell her story. See it for yourself at http://immersive.healthcentral.com/rheumatoid -arthritis/d/LBLN/living-with-ra/.

STIMULATI EXPERIENCE #2:
USE THE *METTA BHAVANA* MEDITATION

Every book I have recently read talks about meditation in some way or another. You have probably been reading about it a lot as well. That's because it works and is changing lives! People who meditate know that it is a practice that is accessible to all, regardless of your religion or spirituality. Meditation goes beyond religion, as it is a direct experience of the mind, and it allows us to feel a deep peace and joy. Shit, who doesn't want that?

Meditation has been proven to have real benefits that can assist in healing. It takes practice, but as you learn to calm your mind and listen to your body, the body will speak its truth, allowing your hidden potential to surface and ultimately having a healing effect. But don't take my word for it. These benefits were first studied in an academic setting by Herbert Benson, MD, at Harvard University. He found that meditation affects physiology, including a decrease in sympathetic nervous system activity; a decrease in heart rate, respiratory rate, and cortisol levels; and an increase in metabolic activity. He also found it promotes better sleep and thinking. People who are anxious about their illnesses can quiet and clear their mind during the highly relaxed state of meditation.[1]

In a 2008 study published in the *Journal of Personality and Social Psychology*, researchers found that the practice of a loving-kindness meditation, similar to the one detailed below, produced increases in daily experiences of positive emotions, which over time led to an increase in developing a purpose in life.[2] And as you've already learned in the last chapter, an increase in satisfaction through finding your purpose reduces depressive symptoms as well as decreases symptoms of illness.

This particular meditation cultivates the emotions that surround loving-kindness for ourselves and for those we are at odds with. It worked wonders for me: Through this deep meditation, I had an *aha* moment that changed the way I felt about my story. I realized *this pain I'm experiencing is a common experience; it does not define me. I'm not alone.*

The idea of cultivating emotions might sound odd: After all, don't emotions just happen? From a Buddhist point of view, that's not the case, and meditation encourages us to take responsibility for our emotional states. Through meditation I learned that emotions are habits we create. If we bring awareness to our emotional life, then we can cultivate the emotions we want to experience and discourage the ones we don't.

Imagine how different you would feel if you encouraged emotions that brought about a sense of calm, love, and well-being. That's what the *Metta Bhavana* is all about. It's a meditation in which we consciously set up the conditions for experiencing the awesomeness of emotions. It is a meditation on happiness, consideration, kindness, and generosity.

Pick a regular time to meditate, and when you do, choose a spot where you can be calm and undistracted. Sit with your feet flat on the floor. You can even lie down in a quiet space where you can turn off as many distractions as possible. Get a little crazy and dim the lights. Or go wild and light a couple of candles. Some people meditate in silence, while others listen to some New Agey tunes or chants. Try recording yourself reading aloud the steps below so you can play it back during your practice and not break your zen by stopping to read.

Take 15 minutes each day, perhaps just after you've awakened (I use my work commute), to practice the following meditation. There are many versions of this meditation, and I have taken some creative license with it. Read the following words slowly and let them sink in so that they become your aspirations. Or have someone you love and trust read to you.

As you breathe, imagine a wave of relaxation sweeping through your body, washing all of your tensions into the earth. Then imagine a wave of energy flowing upward from the earth into your body. Take your awareness into your body and relax your muscles. Let go of any tension in the shoulders, arms, and legs. Relax the muscles in the back of your neck, your jaw, your eyes, and your forehead.

Next take your awareness into your heart, noticing any feelings or emotions that are present. Begin repeating the phrase May I be well,

may I be happy, may I be free from suffering, *and at the same time,*
imagine yourself well and happy. Picture yourself laughing, really laughing.
Notice how this affects your body and mind.

First focus on yourself. Picture yourself now
or how you imagine yourself in the future.

You are free from danger.

You are free from concern.

You are free from physical pain.

You are laughing joyfully.

Feel the love for this happy, laughing, at-ease you.

Stay here for a few minutes.

Next picture three close friends or family members.
See them free from danger.

See them completely free from concern and physical pain.

See them laughing uncontrollably with one another in joy,
their eyes and faces lit up in happiness.

Feel the love for them and the gratefulness for their joy:
It makes you happy, too.

Stay here for a few minutes.

Next picture someone you don't know well but see often:
a cashier, someone who works in your library, a barista.

Picture them free from danger.

Picture them completely free from concern and pain.

Picture them laughing with a large smile, joyfully.

Stay with them for a few minutes.

Next picture someone you have had a fight or issue with.

See them free from danger.

See them free from concern and pain.

Picture them with a huge smile, laughing uncontrollably.

Stay with them in forgiveness and joy for a few minutes.

*Next picture your city. Imagine a white, calming light
coming from your heart or fingertips and spreading to all the
people on the street, into homes, office buildings, and cars.*

*When this light hits them, they smile in joy and laugh,
free from pain or concern.*

*Picture this light spreading to the next town, state,
and now surrounding the world.*

*Feel the love and calmness of this light and the
joy and laughter it brings.*

May all beings,

all breathing things,

all creatures,

all individuals,

all those in sadness and pain,

be free from danger,

be free from mental suffering,

be free from physical suffering.

May they take care and be joyous and happy.

Slowly open your eyes. Be aware of the changes that have taken place in your body and mind, whether those changes are subtle or quite noticeable. Breathe.

STIMULATI MELVIN BRITTON-MILLER:
YOU CAN BE BETTER, AND YOU DESERVE TO HEAL

Stimulati Reverend Melvin Britton-Miller, a life coach and trainer in experiential behavior transformation, taught me a valuable lesson in how I was going to use these truths to write my new story. He taught me that we can learn to push fear aside and believe the statement *my illness is scary, but I can overcome and live life to the fullest.*

Melvin is a New York City community pastor, life coach, and classically trained ballet dancer. He is a graduate of Columbia University as well as the Union Theological Seminary, and he began work as a minister at the Riverside Church. An interesting footnote to Melvin's story is that he happens to be gay. When he first came out, the church where he was working wouldn't allow him to continue to preach. He had a real-life crisis around his belief system; he doubted that he could be a church leader and connected to God because of his sexuality. He stopped working as a reverend and became a motivational coach and

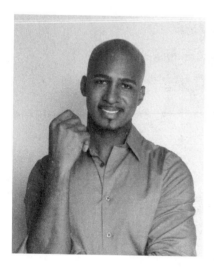

Melvin Britton-Miller

public speaker. Eventually, he returned to the church and his calling. Yet he changed his story completely, and when he did, he learned that anything was possible, including getting married to the man of his dreams in the same church that had fired him. Anything is possible.

Melvin completed his Clinical Pastoral Education training at NYU Langone Medical Center, where he served as a spiritual presence and learned how to work with people who worked at or were treated in a hospital. He's been instrumental in helping thousands of people, from those who are dealing with chronic illness, to those in cognitive care or labor and delivery, to those in the emergency room. It was through this chaplaincy work that he started thinking about the intersection of health, psychology, and religion, and later went back to school for a master's degree in psychology and religion.

Melvin recently told me, "I started looking at the psychological methods of working with people and how they deal with healing. I saw firsthand how we instinctively obey our beliefs. Those beliefs affect your attitude, behaviors, and actions. When you get to the root issue, which is the beliefs that you have, I found that if you can change the beliefs, then you can change the life and, even more important, the experience of life. We're going to live life as we have it until we don't, until we don't have the days on earth anymore. The question becomes, 'What are the beliefs that you're holding that are influencing your experience?'"

Later, Melvin learned to incorporate experiential learning. This is the learning-by-doing approach, and both he and I believe it best allows people to discover how to shift their story. When you are taking part in experiential learning, you actually feel the discovery, and once you feel it, you can't unfeel it: The experience brings about a revelation of knowledge. The Stimulati experiences in this book are inspired by Melvin's teachings.

I met Melvin when I took one of his experiential-learning classes. He reinforced my understanding that I could move on from the past because I can never relive yesterday. In order to move on from your past, you have to stop telling yourself negative things. But first you need to know your thoughts in order to change them. Notice when you are ruminating. Then see if you can push fear aside and turn your ruminations on their head. For example, your story does not have to be *I can't; I'm tired, weak, and in pain.* If you turned that thought into a positive one, you might come up with *my illness is a challenge I can overcome and live life to the fullest. I can be better, and I deserve to heal.*

Melvin told me about a client named Betty who was completely independent for her entire life. But when Betty became ill, she had to receive help from others, and that made her uncomfortable and angry. Melvin taught her that one of the greatest ways you can love a person is to allow them to help you. This idea completely shifted her whole mindset, her understanding of why she was sick, and the people who wanted to help her. Without the negative connotation associated with needing help, she achieved a greater level of openness, forgiveness, vulnerability, and acceptance. Betty was able to make sense of how even in her illness she matters and her illness matters. She changed her story from a bitter, self-righteous person who's sick and not letting anybody help her to a person who can express love through support and openness. It shifted her whole way of being.

I was once working as a staff member at a 4-day seminar, helping to facilitate a class on personal transformation. The goal of the event was to transform negative thoughts to positive ones. An older man came into the room. Louis was much too young to look the way he did. At 65 years old, he'd already had five surgeries on his spinal cord. He walked into the room completely hunched over; his face, his demeanor, and everything about him were painful and heavy. He walked with a cane. He had trouble getting to his seat and he had trouble getting to the bathroom, and he relied on his wife and his cane tremendously.

By the end of the seminar, Louis had released so much emotion by letting go of his negative inner narrative that he came to a point where he was feeling less pain. In fact, he got up, and although he still seemed connected to his wife and others, he didn't need their help anymore. By day 2, Louis was steady enough to walk without holding on to his wife's arm. By day 3, he wasn't using the cane. By day 4, Louis had completely changed his mindset, and he was ready to battle his illness. At the end of the seminar he told me that although he still needed back surgery, he had released so much negative emotion that he was standing up straight. He was still in a lot of pain, but he was ready to do what it took to get to the next step of his life. Louis told me that he felt like 100 pounds had been lifted off of his back. I'm not saying that Louis was cured in one weekend, but I believe that when you release negative emotions while connecting to love, you can jump-start your desire to take control of your health.

According to neuroscientist Alex Korb, PhD, a well-developed thought is like a ski track in the snow. The more you ski down a path, the easier it is to go down that path and not another. This is why it can be so difficult to rewrite your story. But once you've identified the emotions that support your story, you can reprogram how you're feeling about the things you're telling yourself. First replace old narratives with new affirmations, disrupting the negative thoughts circulating in your head and replacing them with positive ones. Melvin taught me how these positive mantras can help me stay in the present. His use of affirmations is the best way I have seen to rewire your thinking. Saying positive statements aloud, saying them to yourself, or writing them down helps retrain habitual thinking. These positive affirmations or mantras reprogram your subconscious to go immediately to *this is something that I can do; there's nothing that I can't manifest or overcome* instead of *I can't*.

For example, Melvin told me a story about a cancer patient he was working with during his residency at Hartford Hospital:

One of the affirmation therapies that I created was called a vision statement. A vision statement starts with a large piece of blank paper. I would say to a patient, "Since you're on this journey, what do you want to call forth? How do you want this journey to be?" One patient told me, "I want the people who I love to forgive me for all that I've done. I want them to know that I love them and that I forgive them. I want to experience a sense of peace."

I had her create a vision statement by writing down on the large paper the affirmation *I am love, forgiveness, and peace.* This became her mantra, and every time she had a chemotherapy session we would put the vision statement up in the room. I had all the nurses, doctors, therapists, as well as her children, sign the vision statement. Their signature meant *we stand with you inside of this, and we see you and we're with you.* The patient realized that she was not alone in this declaration. That positive affirmation carried her all the way through her chemotherapies and her radiation and offered her a sense of hope. On the hardest days, she was able to look at that vision statement and find some sense of peace and hope, even though it was the darkest moment of her life.

One program Melvin started is called You Matter. It combines faith, spirituality, ideology, and history of life. One of the questions it poses is *what is the legacy that you're going to leave with your life?* Melvin sees this question as a moment of declaration and creation. Once you have an answer, then ask yourself, *how do I bring that to the present?* By thinking in this way, you are bringing your future into the present and creating something you can work on today.

I was able to rewrite my story with the affirmation *I accept myself exactly the way I am*. I can call on this affirmation at any time, in any moment when I'm feeling down. It also helps me feel like I am less of a burden to others. In fact, I'm shifting that belief of *I'm a burden, I'm sick, and people have to take care of me. I'm messing up people's lives. Now they have to deal with me* to *I matter because I have goals for my future*.

The coolest part is that science backs up Melvin's teachings. In an experiment published in 2014 in the journal *Medicine & Science in Sports & Exercise*, researchers found that exercisers who said positive mantras to themselves during their routine were able to exercise longer and with less pain. Scientists proposed that exercise-related fatigue was regulated in the brain rather than the muscles. This psychobiological model posits that with the right suggestions, you could convince your brain that you can go farther or harder than it would otherwise allow. The participants who verbally encouraged themselves were able to affect their mind's calculations and stave off fatigue.[3]

We are what we say we are. When researchers have found that psychobiological interventions are beneficial to endurance performance, it makes me think we can convince ourselves that we are capable of anything. What's more, a positive affirmation can make any situation more manageable, even pleasurable.

STIMULATI EXPERIENCE #3:
JUST TAP IT

Another tool that can help rewire your thinking and your nervous system is tapping, a behavior modification therapy gaining acceptance by psychologists and others across the country. Also known as Emotional Freedom Techniques (EFT), tapping is an emotionally based therapeutic tool that is a combination of the best practices of ancient Chinese acupressure and modern psychology. First developed in 1979 by psychologist Roger Callahan, it is meant to interrupt patterns and habits we form deep in the brain that can be related to almost anything: pain, addiction, or mood. Done correctly it can help you get to the root cause of a problem, then help you balance the mind and body in order to change the bad behavior or feeling into one that is more empowering. At one point in my journey, I used tapping so much that I should have had bruises on my chest and forehead. I'm proof it works.

According to Nick Ortner, the bestselling author of *The Tapping Solution*, this practice alleviates stress by disengaging the fight-or-flight response, deactivating the brain's arousal pathways, and reprogramming the brain and body to react differently. Lightly tapping on the meridian end points—the energy channels that carry the vital life force to the organs and other systems of the body and are known to heal the body and block pain—sends a calming response to the body and brain. These meridian points are located primarily on the face: the eyebrow, side of the eye, under the eye, under the nose, and chin. It also requires tapping on the collarbone, under the arm, top of the head, and on the side of the hand.

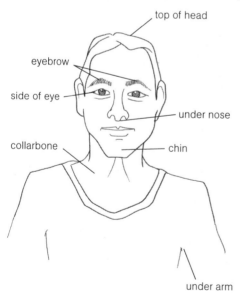

Traditional tapping requires that you imagine your pain, or whatever you are struggling with, and turn that vision into a statement of how you feel about that struggle. Then you end the statement with a positive affirmation. This technique is another type of exposure therapy: You focus on the negative aspects of your experience and then rewrite your story into how you want to experience the same thing differently. Researchers believe that by combining exposure therapy with physical tapping, you can quickly reprogram your brain to turn the negative struggle into a neutral experience so that when it comes up again, the brain does not respond in the same manner. This is why tapping is another tool to bring acceptance and awareness to your current story and show you a path to change it.

You can tap on anything that is bothering you: physical symptoms, emotional upsets, life events in the present or past, future worries, or even limiting beliefs. The process is easy, and the best part is that you can do it on your own. Here's how.

1. Think of a struggle you are currently dealing with. It can be either mental or physical.

2. Create a statement that clearly defines your struggle as part of an affirmation. It could be *I'm suffering and in pain, but it's okay; I still completely accept myself.* Repeat this statement three times as you tap on the side of your hand.

3. Then start tapping. With two fingers, tap five to seven times in a row at the following locations: on the eyebrows, on the sides of the eyes, under the eyes, under the nose, and on the chin. Then tap on your collarbone, under your arm, and on top of your head. As you tap, say a shorter, reminder phrase out loud. This phrase can be something like *this pain.*

4. Take a deep breath and check in with yourself regarding how you feel. Are you less stressed? Are you in less pain? It's likely that you will feel a difference.

5. You can repeat as necessary. However, in the next round, change your statement from the one in step 2 to one that is even more specific and possibly tied to an emotion. For instance, your second statement could be *I'm angry about my back pain, but it's okay; I still completely accept myself.*

STIMULATI EXPERIENCE #4:
TAKE A BREATHER

Are you ready for an easy, anxiety-squashing, happiness-inducing challenge? For the next week, start your day with this three-part exercise, which will help determine your baseline awareness. You can also use this tool when you find yourself upset, flustered, or back in one of the earlier stages of grief that may be surrounding your struggle. This can be a mini meditation to use anytime you start to spiral into an old, self-defeating story. A simple exercise like this allows the space and time to reset your intentions.

This exercise combines three major weapons that combat anxiety, fear, and self-doubt: tapping, positive affirmations, and Tolle's take on a breathing meditation. Start by quickly relaxing your body using the same technique I described to get ready for meditation. Feel your muscles loosen from the top of your head to your toes. Pay close attention to your jaw, you crazy TMJ-ers. Get comfy and then be still. For 1 full minute, feel the air going into your nostrils, and then breathe out through your mouth. Relax a little bit deeper with each breath: Rather than collapsing, simply soften and take that next breath with a little more appreciation for the air that is keeping you alive. It might take five breaths for you to become fully engaged, but when you do this type of mindful breathing, you can't possibly concentrate on your breath and your worries at the same time. Remember, deep breath in through your nose, feeling it come in those nostrils, then blow it out of your mouth. Focus your thoughts on how the air feels.

Next do two rounds of tapping as described above. Finally, recite one affirmation three times in the mirror. For this exercise, try the following: *This moment is all that exists; I don't need to worry about the rest. All is okay.*

The Purpose of Doubts

Accepting the truth doesn't mean that you will not have doubts or that you won't bump up against brand-spanking-new obstacles as your new story unfolds. Remember my story about working on Wall Street as a specialist trader after I graduated from college? The truth is that although I like to boast about it, I disliked that job. It was hard for me physically because I had to stand up all day, I didn't like my environment, and because I wasn't loving the work, I made lots of mistakes. One day I had one of the largest trades on the American Stock Exchange: Millions of dollars had traded instantly, and everyone on the floor was frantic, trying to understand what was happening. Was it a merger, a takeover? What was happening in the market?! Whoops, sorry guys, none of the above. I electronically traded the wrong stock and in seconds lost millions of dollars. I went completely numb with fear and shock. When I realized what I had done, I knew I was going down fast. This mistake had major consequences: It impacted my career, my employer, my coworkers, the company I was trading, and potentially the general public. I realized that I had a small window of opportunity to fix it, so I left my post and went to talk with everyone who had participated in my trade. I convinced each trader to forgive the trade and send it to the "DK" room, where all "Don't Know" trades go to die. The tragedy was averted, the situation corrected. But I realized I couldn't take this roller coaster of a career. My mistake was the wake-up call I needed, and I started looking for a new job the next day.

Choosing to do something else was not easy. I had studied finance in college. I had told everybody that the job I had was my goal, and because I was able to secure it, I was respected. Plus, I made a lot of money (or so I thought at the time), and being a trader fit my macho story perfectly. Once I made the decision to leave, the negative voice in my head started to speak up: *You're not good enough to find another job. What if you don't like the new job either? You invested so much time in your education, in this job, and you're going to change now?*

The self-doubt continued until I landed at a publicly traded start-up (it was the '90s, after all) in health technology that I actually had traded at my last job. I knew more about that company than any of the other applicants, so they put me into business development and sales. I had my own desk, a comfortable chair, and the flexibility to go to the doctor when I needed to. The company's advertisements featured a cute dog with the word *therapy* on its name tag—this could not be any more opposite from the dogfight I had just left on Wall Street. Immediately, my stress level lowered. I lost weight. The pain in my joints went down, and I found flow at work. I began to excel. I became the number one salesperson in a short time. From there, I went on to do business development for the company that purchased us, called WebMD, long before it went public. After we had the IPO, I left to help develop another company in that same realm, called Everyday Health. With each new job I overcame my own doubts, found meaning in what I was doing, and created a story that eventually allowed me to uncover my purpose and financial freedom. Remember, living a purposeful life will make you stronger, better, and bolder.

When your mind raises doubts, consider it to be your signal to change your story. You know a doubt in your body through the uneasy feeling it creates before you ever recognize it in your mind. Be aware of that gut feeling and trust it!

THOUGHT IGNITER
Consider this: Your story points to your purpose.

CHAPTER 3

REPROGRAMMING YOUR SHAME, ANGER, AND RESENTMENT

THOUGHT IGNITER:

Oh, what the fuck, do whatever it takes!

My gut reaction to the word *victim* is to shudder and think that's not something I ever want to be. Shit, the word has such a negative connotation that we often use it as a derogatory statement to hurt someone in an argument. After all, with synonyms like *loser, prey, stooge, dupe, sucker, quarry, fool, fall guy,* and *chump,* who would ever admit to being or wanting to be a victim? Yet it's easy to feel like you are a victim when you are facing a chronic illness or some other trauma. You may think that you're sick for some karmic reason. You may think that you deserve your plight and should learn to live with it, because feeling better is not possible. You may feel that you are receiving some kind of cosmic punishment, that you were responsible for your condition because you are a bad person or have treated others poorly. If you are in survival mode, you might even believe that your suffering is normal.

I've discovered that so many chronically ill people find comfort in their despair when they are in survival mode. I know this because I was there. My pain made it easy for me to not face the hard truth and not to try or even follow through on the recommendations of experts that might have made me feel better. The truth was, I needed to make changes and work harder to be at my best and heal. But that ain't easy! And when I was challenged, it was much easier to place blame on my illness and my pain than to be bold and take action to make my life better. So I grew accustomed to feeling bad and misconstrued, as I know many do, how I was feeling as normal. I identified with a baseline where even a change for the better was awkward and uncomfortable.

It may have been easy for you to go down the rabbit hole of self-loathing. Oh, and believe me, I did. In my avoidance I lived in the warm blanket of shame. It's like waking up on a cold morning when you're comfortable and still groggy in bed, and for those first few moments, you think you would be happiest if you stayed there all day. It's hard to get out of bed, move into the cold air, and face challenges. But you know you have to leave your protected environment or life is going to pass you by. If you don't get up, you inevitably shame yourself for lying there and wasting your time. Eventually you won't be tired, and the warm blanket will feel more like a restraint than a respite.

When you don't feel well or believe that you don't deserve the necessary treatments that will make you feel better or even happy, self-destructive feelings become your shame. These are the *not enough* feelings that signal that you are in survival mode. Yet they do not have to be your story. As we learned in the last chapter, each of us is whole and complete the way we are right now. Please accept this for what it is. No matter what is wrong with you, you are at the perfect place at the perfect time. There is far more to you than the dysfunction or function of your mind or body. After all, you love your best friends for all of their flaws: Why not treat yourself the same way?

In this chapter, you will learn how to disrupt guilt and shame, two bone-crushing emotions that are 100 percent okay to have but likely are holding you back from healing. You don't need to punish yourself anymore. You are not a victim, and you can be healthy. The secret is to turn your vulnerability on its head, making it your secret weapon instead of a weakness.

THE MANY LAYERS OF SHAME

Shame on you, shame! Shame is a sense of failure, hurt, or harm; it's the emotion that comes up when we feel that we've done something wrong to others or ourselves. At its core, shame is secretive: We rarely share our shame with others. The burden of shame is the belief that if this secret should ever get out, or if people should ever uncover this ugly piece of your story, then they will think less of you. Shame often looks like *I'm bad because I'm ill* or *I'm ill because I'm bad.*

Ever shut down and tune out when it comes to doing something or talking about yourself? You probably have shame to thank for that. When shame makes you shut down and tune out, it creates stress, despair, loneliness, and disconnection, and it's often the emotional driver of the chronically ill. It sets the tone for everything you do regarding decision making for your care, your relationships, and more. For example, I was lying to everyone I met out of shame, and that drove the emotions I allowed myself to feel.

When I hid in the shadows of shame, my denial, depression, and fear about my illness were the catalysts that helped me create a facade. The motorcycle accident that never happened could explain my disabilities rather than admitting to people that I was sick. A motorcycle accident doesn't relapse; a motorcycle accident doesn't get worse with time; a motorcycle accident wouldn't lead people to ask if I was contagious. A motorcycle accident could happen—even to a good person. So I would tell this lie when I applied for a job or when I went out on dates with new women. It was my shield, but it was so strong that it prevented me from getting close to anyone. My lack of vulnerability and the disconnection that my lies created left me lonely, sad, and sick. No one really knew me outside of my immediate family.

The underlying belief about shame is *my body doesn't matter; I don't matter. I'm not worthy, and so my body's not worthy for anyone to take the time to make it better.* For example, when someone gains weight and the weight won't go away, shame becomes his codependent coping mechanism. Until you're able to change your story, the healthiness of your body is an extension of the healthiness of your story.

Social media can be shame's biggest ally. Shame on you, social media! It produces a negative self-image and disconnection. On social media, everyone appears happier than you, richer than you, more beautiful than you. You don't see the mundaneness of life, and it gives us all a warped view of what life is like. When we're not feeling enough to begin with, this has a tendency to make us feel like we have even less. In response, we manufacture a false story of our own happiness, but again, living within a lie leaves you living without any vulnerability.

Social media will also happily hand you the trigger for your shame. One of my favorite ways to get through a sleepless night was stalking my ex-girlfriend's boyfriend on Facebook. I know, I know—that is an obvious no-no. But of course I would find what I was looking for, as all things hold the meaning you give them: pictures of them together "in love" and "happy" in some awesome location. I'd spiral into inadequacy and *not enough-ness* around the loss of the relationship, then shame myself for not only the relationship's ending but also for Facebook stalking them. Now I know better, and I recommend taking regular vacations from social media and treating it like a loaded gun: with caution.

Fear is an emotion associated with shame; it comes along for the ride. There is the fear of losing social standing or being humiliated, and if you're sick, there may be a real fear of death, maybe for some perceived wrong you did. My old story was that I couldn't be loved until I got better. I was afraid that someone would discover my inadequacies and think less of me. I was embarrassed about the first impression I presented to new people when they saw me walk. I feared my limitations would never be resolved.

There's also a cycle of shame and anger: Shame causes anger, and anger causes shame. It doesn't matter where you are in the cycle, because both emotions can make you feel like a victim, trapping you in your illness and creating a cuckoo, anxious mind. Victims use anger as a wall against vulnerability, leaving them stuck and alone, believing that nothing can be done.

There is another sense of shame that is closely related to guilt. It is the part of shame that is associated with not wanting to be a burden on our family, our friends, and even our doctors and professional caretakers. It manifests when you think, *my illness is a burden on someone else.* This burden can be especially hard if you have previously been self-sufficient: In that moment when you need people the most, you don't know how to ask for help. I felt this burden when it became clear that even with their best intentions, my parents were getting tired of taking me from one hospital to another.

Once I was able to let go of the guilt, anger, and shame that had become such a large part of my illness, I could break free from my survival mode and actually allow people to give me support and love. As I let more people into my life and practiced this, I became less fearful and more vulnerable. I was no longer a victim of my illness.

Whoa, I know that is big, confusing, and overwhelming when you think of it as a whole. *Is it possible to let go? Wake up and presto, your shame is gone?* I'm an optimist, but I will tell you that it takes work, and if you do the work, you can get there. In fact, you've already started tossing off your shame. Each chapter of this book builds on itself: recognizing your old, distracting story; changing your beliefs by creating a new, bolder one that is aligned with the truth; and then using tools like meditation and tapping to calm yourself and reprogram your fears, the shame and anger will no longer have a place to camp out in your mind. Trust me on this. Keep doing the work and you will get there, too.

This is exactly how I learned to move on from being stuck in my past stories and create an awesome current story built around what I want for the future.

Stimulati Melvin Britton-Miller was integral in helping me release my old story and its heavy burden of shame. Along with that, I released 40 pounds of weight, which allowed me to be much more comfortable in my own body, both figuratively and literally. I realized I was holding on to the heaviness in my heart that was literally keeping me heavy physically. It was at this same time that my body began to heal. Releasing anger and shame lowers stress in both the body and the mind, and lower

---

SELF-HELP ALERT: When you see the limitlessness of the future, you can transform from victim to hero and take responsibility for your mindset and health. Heroes inspire others by the actions their story allows them to take. You can craft a new story of strength and an ability to overcome the odds. It is 100 percent possible, and when you do so, your example can inspire others, creating a domino effect that positively impacts the world.

stress levels, once again, have been clearly shown to reduce the inflammation that causes pain, weight gain, and low energy.

You, my friend, are no victim! You are ready to start using a super-powered Thought Igniter I learned from a Momentum Education class. It's called the *Oh, what the fuck, do whatever it takes!* reaction. Try saying this phrase out loud five times. Now try again, and this time, really mean it. Sing it: *Oooooh, what the fuuuuck, doooo whateeeever it taaaakes!*

Oh, what the fuck is letting go of everything that might be holding you back: fear, shame, guilt. *Do whatever it takes* is part of an unstoppable you. This idea goes beyond an affirmation; it's a declaration. Declare that you will not hold yourself back from getting stronger, better, or bolder. That you will let go of the guilt, shame, and fear and allow yourself to do whatever it takes to heal. Make this declaration at the moment you've convinced yourself not to go to physical therapy or the gym, and push yourself to go. Make this declaration at the moment you find yourself not wanting to be vulnerable or ask for help from the people whom you truly love. Make this declaration when fear creeps up and tells you that you can't do something—because you can.

WHEN SANDRA LET GO OF SHAME, SHE LOST 150 POUNDS

Melvin shared a story of a woman he helped to release the shame she was carrying about her weight so that she could create a different story. Here's what he told me.

Sandra was a mentee of mine, a life coach I'd trained. She was talented, but her weight posed a real challenge, and I saw it as a barrier to her success. One day I decided I had to have a conversation with her about it, even though I knew it would be a difficult conversation to have. I told her, "If you ever want to coach professionally, if you ever want to lead a room and train a room, you're going to have to take care of your weight. When people look at you, your weight becomes a distraction."

In that 5-minute conversation, we cried together, and it was in that moment that she made a choice to matter in a different way than she had before. It was her choice to investigate how she could lose weight most effectively, and she chose to have lap band surgery instead of try another diet and feel bad about herself when it didn't work. The surgery allowed her to become a completely different person. Sandra lost 150 pounds, but more importantly, she has kept the weight off by diligently monitoring her eating. Now she is coaching and has answered her life's call. Acknowledging her purpose and acknowledging what it would take to fulfill her purpose gave her the where-withal to have a huge transformation. It not only empowered her to stand in front of a room but also helped her tell a story that compels and moves people and is 100 percent authentic.

STIMULATI DAVID STEINDL-RAST: GRATEFULNESS IS AN ANTIDOTE TO FEAR

Brother David Steindl-Rast believes that when you are grateful, you cannot be fearful. Without fear, you are more willing to share. Sharing and contribution lead to purpose.

Brother David was born in 1926 in Vienna, Austria. He studied art, anthropology, and psychology, receiving an MA from the Academy of Fine Arts Vienna and a PhD from the University of Vienna. In 1953, he joined the Mount Saviour Monastery Community in New York, becoming a Benedictine monk. He's the cofounder of Gratefulness.org, and he was one of the first Roman Catholics to participate in Buddhist-Christian dialogue. Brother David believes that gratefulness comes when you are given something of great value, but this type of gratefulness happens only once in a while. Grateful living is something we can have all the time. We can live gratefully by becoming more aware that every moment is a gift and that we have no way of knowing that there will be another moment like it given to us. Within this moment is an opportunity, and if we avail ourselves of the opportunity, moment by moment, we can be grateful for this gift. When bad things happen—and they will—we do not have to be grateful for those moments, but we can see them as passing moments, rise to the occasion, and respond appropriately. Nothing is as bad as it seems if you believe that the next moment holds the promise to be better.

Now, let's be honest: Is this easy to do? No, it is not. However, it gets easier with practice. Just being aware and trying to be more grateful will move you in the right direction. I think of this concept as less of an instruction and more of a reminder to not take what is good in my life— such as my new puppy, my son, my family and friends, writing this book—for granted and to be optimistic about the possibilities that may wash ashore tomorrow.

The Path of Forgiveness

Releasing shame and fear allowed me to dump my emotional burden, and I could finally be the man I wanted to be, more at ease and more confident, because I was making decisions from a place of strength rather than weakness. The next step was to forgive myself for creating my defeatist story in the first place. I forgave myself for having the feelings of shame, guilt, and anger that I was using to keep others at bay.

There will be times when your pain or suffering doesn't involve anyone else and the only person you have to forgive is yourself. Think of it as cleaning the slate. You are lightening your load so that you can actually do what you want to do and be as happy as you can be. And if you are anything like me, start by forgiving yourself for wanting to be perfect. The truth is, the best we can be is perfectly imperfect.

We're all a little fucked up, and so what? Even Superman had his kryptonite. As long as you make an effort, you don't have to beat yourself up, and you can forgive yourself and start to move forward.

My forgiveness mantra is *I'm not perfect, and I accept myself for being exactly who I am. I am forgiven. I am pretty damn good.* Say this enough and you will rewire the beliefs your stories are built on.

Next figure out who else you want to forgive. There might be instances when you feel someone has wronged you and you will want to forgive them so that you can release your shame. It might involve your parents or others who influenced your childhood, such as a grandparent or a sibling. We form strong impressions about how life works during the ages of 3 to 7 years old, and our perceptions of events during these years is often melded into our story.

Forgiving these people is a crucial step for healing: If you don't forgive others, regardless of their intentions, you cannot release the negative emotions holding you back from optimal health. The reason is that forgiveness is personal. It is for you and you alone, regardless of whomever you need to forgive. Even though your suffering may be connected to another person, it's your experience and your feelings. It's your pain to let go and not someone else's. You don't have to tell someone you forgive them, and I am not asking you to forget anything or absolve anyone of their actions. In fact, sometimes you may have to remove yourself from their circle of influence. I am asking that you let shit go because it is good for you and only you. When you remove anger and forgive, it is like a lead weight has been lifted off of your shoulders and you can breathe again.

We can forgive somebody without ever uttering a word to them. When you are alone in a quiet, safe place, try saying something like this out loud (tailoring it to your situation): *You hurt me. Who treats a child like that? I still get emotional when I think of you exploding with rage and hurling a wine bottle at the wall. But I know you are human and have flaws like us all, and although I don't forget, I am no longer carrying the burden of that pain. I am letting it go for myself, because it is in the past. I forgive you and accept you for being imperfect.*

You can actually tell the person that you are forgiving them, but remember, forgiveness is for you. Don't expect them to respond in any particular way or you will likely be disappointed.

BURN, BABY, BURN

Melvin taught me an amazing technique for achieving forgiveness and letting go of shame and guilt that has nothing to do with the person who has harmed you and everything to do with you as an individual. Again, you don't need to involve the other person in order to heal: Forgiveness starts with you.

This simple exercise is both ritualistic and symbolic. It's about making the decision to let go and create a new story. Write down all the things that you feel upset about, feel shame and guilt about, and want to get over and forgive. Write each one down on separate small pieces of paper. Then get a small metal trash can or make a fire in your fireplace or outdoor fire pit. Read each piece of paper out loud and then rip it in pieces and toss it into the fire. As they burn away, realize you are letting them go. Last, say aloud, *I have let this go.*

When I did this ritual for the first time, I had had enough of my stories. I was exhausted from my lies around my illness and motorcycle accidents as well as the macho stories and the belief that I had to still act like the tough guy of my youth. I realized it wasn't working: The burden I was carrying was too great. Oprah would be proud of me: It was an aha moment, and once I got there, I realized that this ritual opened me up to a lot of possibilities for letting go psychologically and emotionally. It is all about small realizations that lead to a much bigger understanding.

Now I am a different kind of tough guy, one who burns little pieces of paper when I'm alone in the dim lights of my bedroom with the details of my shame written on them. I can do that because my story now is that there isn't anything I can't do, and I accept the shit out of myself.

You can do this ritual as many times as you need, because old habits of shame and guilt tend to stick around. It's likely you will need reinforcement, but I am betting you will immediately begin to feel lighter and find new doors to open. You have to keep making the same choice over and over again to let these negative emotions go. If they do reappear, you can be aware of these feelings and then release them again. Before you know it, they will be gone for good.

STIMULATI BRENT BAUM:
RELEASING YOUR OLD STORY

Brent Baum, a trauma specialist and real McCoy energy healer in Arizona, taught me that while we can't change the past, we can change the way we perceive the present and think about the future. I know that is some heavy stuff. The Bauminator, as I call him, works with positive visualization and memory resolution. I found Brent through research I was doing on energy healing and went to Arizona to work with him.

I've seen him multiple times and spent hours working through a number of different experiences.

The Bauminator's life story covers every aspect of healing. He first studied to be a Catholic priest but became frustrated that the people who came to him for healing kept reliving the same traumatic events. Their progress wasn't an issue of willpower or dependent on whether they were living a moral life; it seemed to be more about where they were stuck subconsciously.

He left the priesthood and became a licensed addiction counselor. But as before, week after week people would come in for treatment and repeat the same patterns: They were not getting better. They were stuck in a loop, repeating the same feelings and the same event without even realizing it.

About that time, Brent came across the work of a psychologist from New Zealand named David Grove who believed in empowering people to heal themselves. Grove discovered that we pause our consciousness, or, in other words, tune out as we're being overwhelmed by something. That feeling of being overwhelmed is then stored in both the mind and the body, and if we don't address it, we're destined to relive that event forever. Brent saw the validity in Grove's argument and felt it explained a lot about what was happening to the people who came for treatment, whether they were relapsing into drug abuse or reliving painful events with family members.

Brent realized that much of the pain we experience can be related to either emotionally or physically painful memories, much like the brain-body connection of post-traumatic stress disorder we discussed in Chapter 1. By the early 1990s, Brent discovered that the majority of migraine patients who came for treatment were often reliving experiences of an original migraine event. The same held true for panic attacks. Neck and back pain could often be traced to a car accident or another traumatic event, even if they were in the distant past. Even allergies were often linked to traumatic events: When the body couldn't handle emotionally what was going on, it captured a reaction to whatever environmental trigger was around at the time of the event.

His mother was an empath and could feel when her children were in accidents and had injuries. Brent found that he had similar abilities and started using this gift to determine effective techniques for resolving memory. At an early age, he realized that he had an intuitive power and an ability to actually feel and work with energy, meaning the unseen human energy that we all possess. He believes that through the combined use of energy healing and memory resolution, we can reframe past negative memories so that we can move forward in a more positive light and let old things go. When we do, we can release much of the blocks and stresses within our body, reduce pain, and knock out depression.

Based on Grove's premise, Brent developed a technique that identifies where the body holds and stores memory. He believes that while you can't undo a death or a traumatic event, you can teach the body to rewrite or rescript that event so that we can get unstuck from the moment when consciousness freezes and we tune out of awareness.

Brent taught me that every day, we cycle in and out of old memories 15 to 50 times per hour. Try to follow yourself through a single hour and see how many times your attention shifts. Sometimes this shift in attention produces anxiety. We all have memories that we wish were different.

In Brent's own words,

We know from brain research using single-photon emission computed tomography (SPECT) scanners that your brain doesn't know the difference between the original event and the memory of the event. We go back into the same brain wave pattern and the same state of physiological distress as the original event. The positive ones, of course, are not a problem; that's how we motivate ourselves and move through our day. The negative ones, however—you can hook into the physiology of a past event. The stress and trauma create self-hypnotic moments that are both automatic and subconscious. When that occurs, you're going to have an automatic fight, flight, freeze reaction. Adrenaline will go up, and when the adrenaline rises, your thymus cell production and your immunity will drop. When that's happening many times per hour, we end up with an increase in autoimmune disorders. When we overproduce adrenaline, we push too hard, and we get sick.

If memory, as the neurophysiologists are telling us, is stored in a hologram-like manner, then even a fragment of a memory might be stored energetically. A fragment of a memory has the capacity to resurrect the whole thing. If a fragment remains in the system, then the whole thing can present itself as a pain syndrome, and we know that is phantom pain, where even if you lose a limb or an organ, you can still feel it—pain and all.

Brent's therapies were influential in reframing some of my negative past beliefs. He showed me how I could let go of them and gain self-awareness so I could start to change my life. Brent's work is a fusion of body psychology, energy psychology, and color psychology, because as the Bauminator says, "Color is an infinite language and is not limited like words." He taught me how to reframe memories using color and how to create a story for the future that moved me forward into better health.

Working with Brent, I would visualize a memory but change the story to something lovable, joyous, or nurturing. I would frame it in the color that this new feeling brought to mind and send that color feeling through my body to prove to my body that I could create safety and that I was no longer in that moment. He calls it emotional reframing and has used it to prevent addicts from relapse as well as to relieve both mental and physical pain.

First I learned to discharge the original frozen moment so I could get unstuck. One experience we worked on involved my father, who had a bit of a temper (I love you, Dad). I was often in a state of high alert. Brent helped me realize that part of my story was that trying to please my father to ensure calm created anxiety in me.

Then Brent worked with me to reframe the relationship with my father in a specific color. We chose green because it was the color that immediately came up for me. We created a visualization and did energy work around what it would be like, and what I would be like, if I were my father. We explored how I would act toward my own son and what my dad would act like. Then we reframed this ideal as if it were real in a green energy field. Very meta, I know, but it worked. During my meditation on this new vision, my entire body was filled with green energy. In my conscious mind I became *green dad*, who is grounded, healing, helping, and happy. I only have to think of those feelings and color when I'm interacting with my son, my girlfriend, and even my father to alleviate anxiety, resentment, or pain.

If you do this technique 50 times over a month or two, each time reframing the new scene the same way, you start to send a feeling of safety to the subconscious mind. Linguistic studies have shown that when you hear something repeated 50 times, it generally goes into the subconscious. Brent said, "I encourage people to do 50 breaths when they reframe a memory, to move that solution through the body 50 times to anchor it in."

I once had an experience with Brent that freaked me out a little but made me a believer in the existence and power of the energy around us. Brent and I were working together, and I brought my phone into the treatment room. The phone was in a bag next to me. We were working on some pain in my feet. I was going to have surgery, and the pain went all the way up

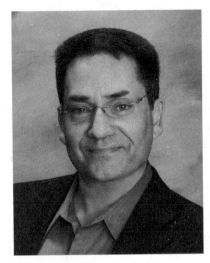

Brent Baum, my favorite trauma specialist and energy healer.

into my ankles. He put me into a trance state, and he identified that the pain was connected to a specific memory that involved my mother and me when I was a young boy. The memory was innocent enough: We were walking through a grocery store and I was complaining about my feet hurting. In her matter-of-fact way, my mother told me to suck it up and stop complaining (I paraphrase). As an adult, I realize that I'd probably react the same way with my son; it's not a huge issue in the grand scheme, but we never know what children will capture as painful.

Brent and I started working to release that memory. We colored the new memory in royal blue and reframed the story in a way that resolved the issue. In my re-creation, my mom stopped, coddled me a little, and focused on resolving my issue. In essence, we turned the memory from one of isolation to one of togetherness. Afterward, the pain in my feet was gone. To this day, I haven't had the surgery.

Yet the truly amazing part of the story occurred a minute later. As I was walking out of his office into the courtyard, my mother called me on my mobile phone. She asked incredulously who I was talking to a few moments ago. Somehow, during our session, my phone had dialed her, and she had listened in to my session. I don't know what happened exactly. Through the power of intention and energy, shit happens. And that is evidence enough for me that there is more to what we're putting out there than we can possibly fathom. Again, anything is possible.

For more information about Brent or to follow one of his guided meditations, visit his website Healingdimensions.com. It has CD and MP3 access, and his latest videos explain his approach.

STIMULATI EXPERIENCE #6:
COLOR FRAMING YOUR STRONGER, BETTER, BOLDER SELF

Take a moment to relax. You have made it this far, so you are doing great. Sit in a comfortable chair or lie down. Uncross your arms and legs and let the tension slip out of your body, starting at the top of your head and moving down to the bottom of your feet. Just relax. Read the following visualization and then try it on for size.

Close your eyes and visualize something from your past that has been causing you pain, concern, worry, or anxiety. Picture yourself in this scene. What is happening? What does it sound like? Who is there with you? What color do you associate with this scene?

Experience this scenario in all of its pain. Now I want you to make it black and white, turn down the volume so you can't hear anything, and shrink the image. Picture a big-screen TV and see this image of pain in a small gray box in the right-hand corner.

Now focus on the full-size screen, the opposite of this picture.
On the bigger screen, you are WHOLE, HEALTHY,
AND LIVING WITHOUT FEAR!
You are wearing clothes that make you feel confident. You are stronger,
better, and bolder. You can manifest anything.

Tell yourself this three times with gusto. Now what new colors
do you see? Green? Blue? Take the color from that reframed
experience and picture it running through your body and bursting out of
your head and fingers and filling everything you can see.
Feel the power of this new comforting, strong, and empowering color and
scene. Picture that new stronger, better, bolder you kicking that
small gray square from the right-hand corner, sending it far off into the
distance until it becomes a small dot and disappears.
All that is left is YOU. Strong, bold, and beautiful.

Open your eyes and stretch your hands and arms up over your head. While still thinking of this color and new image of yourself, repeat again, *Oh, what the fuck, do whatever it takes!* After all, why not? You're worth it, baby!

STIMULATI BRENÉ BROWN:
THE POWER OF VULNERABILITY

Brené Brown, PhD, is a bestselling author and research professor at the University of Houston graduate college of social work. Her groundbreaking TED Talk and books changed my life, which is why I consider her a Stimulati. You can access her talk on vulnerability at www.ted.com/talks/brene_brown_on_vulnerability.

Dr. Brown defines shame as the fear of disconnection. It begs the question, is there something about me that if people knew it or saw it, I would no longer be worthy of connection? This idea of adopting worthiness, which we'll get back to later in the book, is a powerful tool to get rid of shame.

In her research, Dr. Brown found that those who felt most worthy lived lives of courage, compassion, and connection. A sense of courage didn't mean being brave but instead telling your story with your whole heart. I understand this to mean that we can have the courage to be imperfect if we can be compassionate to ourselves and others. With compassion, we can connect more authentically to others because we are being true to ourselves as we are right now.

Dr. Brown also believes that vulnerability is an asset: She defines it as the ability to take risks for yourself and, in relationships, to stop controlling and predicting. In short, in order to release shame, you have to get yourself out of survival mode. When I was in survival mode, I was numb to all of my emotions, not only painful ones of shame and guilt but also the good ones. In order to become vulnerable, I had to learn to open myself to the full range of emotions. I was able to do this by being bold.

For example, for many years, every time I felt anger, fear, concern, or worry, I would visualize myself literally pushing all of those emotions down into my feet (it's not surprising that my illness affected my legs most!). Or I would visualize a snowplow removing them so all I could imagine was white space. Later, I realized that instead of hiding and pushing away these emotions and denying their existence, I had to be bold and let them come up and be experienced and communicated, no matter how painful they were, in order for me to let them go, feel better, and truly connect with people. Sitting with your emotions instead of stifling them, letting yourself experience them fully with vulnerability, and acting on them despite fear is not complicated, but it takes courage.

STIMULATI EXPERIENCE #7:
GAINING THE POWER OF VULNERABILITY

Speaking of courage, this exercise is going to take some, but if you've gotten this far, I know you have it. I'm going to show you how to break whatever is left of your survival mode. You will call some people and ask for help or support. Let your friends and family know that they can support you, that you are now being vulnerable enough to let people know that you don't have to heal on your own. The most obvious choices are those you're closest to in your life whom you've been holding at arm's length.

A specific ask could be *I never told you this before, but I need your love, support, and help. Before I felt like I was a burden, and I want to release that feeling. I can't do this alone. I need you. And I will be there for you. I love you.*

Call three people and have this vulnerable conversation this week.

THE POWER OF COMMUNITY: JOIN A GROUP

According to Melvin, while living a purposeful life will make you stronger, better, and bolder, sometimes we need a helping hand to show us the way. He is a big proponent of group work, and so am I. In his own words, "Breaking the hold of the secret of shame is one of the majestic moments of group work. If people take the time to reach into the life of another human being who is going through the same experience, that causes a deep sense of freedom, relief, and forgiveness. You recognize 'Oh, I'm not by myself. I'm not alone in this. Other people have this shame and guilt and these feelings too. I thought I was the only one.' If people could share and open up with one another through vulnerability, through exercises, through experiences, then they begin to recognize that we're not so different. We may have different lives, but we have the same kinds of lives. We don't have the same psyche, but we have the same kind of psyche."

THOUGHT IGNITER

If you are love, there's no way you can't be loved.
Vulnerability will provide the proof.

CHAPTER 4

GETTING FROM LOVESICK TO LOVE

THOUGHT IGNITER:

Your task is not to seek for love, but merely to seek and find all the barriers within yourself that you have built against it.

—*Unknown*

Lucy Lou was my blue-eyed Kryptonite. We first met while self-helping at a leadership course in New York City. I can still remember the first time we made eye contact: My mind went blank for a moment just looking at her. We were drawn to each other as if we were meant for something more, and we were.

We became close friends and each other's greatest support over the course of the 6-month training and lovers after that. I couldn't imagine my life without her. In fact, doing so created some anxiety. I felt butterflies in my stomach every time I saw her. I had an overwhelming desire to care for her and to make her happy. She could melt me with a look or make me laugh with a sharp comment. We spoke for hours a day and shared every intimate detail about our lives.

Eventually, I bought a ring and waited for the right moment. I was smitten and therefore ignored and rationalized all the red flags and glaring issues we had. So it strikes me as no coincidence that while I was first drafting this chapter, I was experiencing a major knock-you-to-your-knees, think-about-nothing-else, go-through-all-stages-of grief lovesickness. Lucy and I had just broken up. The right moment had never come.

I was feeling physically terrible, even though there was nothing out of the ordinary happening with my health. It wasn't until I was writing that I realized I was relapsing because of my lovesickness!

My symptoms were very much the same as when I was dealing with the worst parts of my illness: lack of energy, lack of self-confidence, depression, and increased anxiety. I was neglecting loving myself: I allowed myself to wallow in a feeling of inadequacy that led to less self-care, I wasn't exercising, and I was making lots of bad food choices. I had a flare of my physical issues, my limp was more pronounced, and my old symptoms started up: stiffness, spasticity in my legs, and pain. There was a sense of unworthiness, low self-esteem, and a general malaise. I lost my zest for life; I was spending too much time and energy obsessing about her, while also feeling sorry for and shaming myself. Oh, and the best one: wondering whom she was being intimate with now that I was out of the picture. I felt like I drank 10 cups of bad coffee and lost my puppy each day, and I was sure that the breakup was my fault: If I had done some things differently, I could have pleased her. If only I was . . . better.

Although my lovesickness was ALL mental and the story I created was one centered on my not being able to make a relationship work (my old, unworthy *I can't be loved* story was fiercely triggered, and as many of you know, that story hurts!), all of my physical symptoms were real. Worst of all, my grief started a different cycle. When I put my own needs on hold, I wasn't able to give the best of myself to those most important to me, like my son, Aidan, and my best friend and sister, Pam, and I watched from the sidelines as those relationships suffered.

My lovesickness progressed when I started to blame my ex. I went into victim mode. I told myself we broke up because she had no capacity for me; she couldn't love me; she must have been cheating; she was to blame for my bad mood and returning symptoms—she made me feel this way. But through writing this book and being aware and honest about how I was feeling, I was able to step back and ask myself if my poor health was caused by her, the relationship, or the resulting breakup. Logically, I knew the answer was NO! My downward slide was due to the situation I created, a combination of self-neglect, a trigger of inadequacy, a tremor in my sense of love, and some pesky rejection-induced neurotransmitting chemicals in my brain. In this situation, my reality reverted to sickness. Through my emotional and mental turmoil, I made myself physically sick.

Once I recognized that only I was responsible for the way I was feeling, I got myself back on track. I took a hard look at myself and my situation: I decided to accept that I felt that way for a reason and it was okay, but that I was creating that story and it was time to take responsibility for my part, forgive any perceived hurts, and move on. Sometimes you have to focus on those who make you feel best, even if it feels like loss or failure. My real story is and always was that I am confident and calm and that things always work out. I learned I could live this story after my days on Wall Street, but remembering it is not always easy. After the breakup, making the switch required awareness, conscious effort, and choice. I had to choose a new story of adequacy and strength and reinforce it with the tools in this book, sometimes a few times per day. Then I was in a better place to tend to my most fulfilling relationships.

What if our struggle, our guilt, and our shame are a form of lovesickness for ourselves? You don't have to go through a traumatic breakup to be lovesick! If you are not loving yourself, you may be experiencing the same emotions that create illness as those associated with the lovesickness after a relationship breaks up. After all, our closest relationship and the one in which we spend vastly more time in is the one we have with ourselves.

In the end, I realized we were indeed meant for something more, and we achieved it. The realizations and lessons we learned from that relationship and the resulting breakup have been invaluable. The good times we had are cherished, and most importantly, I learned I am love and can give it freely to myself and others—no matter what.

STIMULATI JORJA RIVERO: CHOOSING SELF-LOVE

It's hard to have the energy, motivation, and passion to find our purpose or to make positive changes to our health, life, or situation when our self-worth and self-esteem are running on empty. Unfortunately, this is the human default setting. We judge ourselves all the time; we are our

---

SELF-HELP ALERT: Once you've released the burden of shame and guilt, you can continue on your journey to find your purpose by cultivating a new kind of love and appreciation for yourself. In this chapter, you'll learn that we decide what we create, who we are, and how we feel. With self-love, you have the courage to be accepting and nonjudgmental, allowing space to make the best decisions. From here, you begin to create a new reality, where you can start thinking about the future and what your life can be. It starts by filling your own cup first, knowing that you are more than adequate and worthy of having health and happiness.

---

biggest and worst critics. No matter what we do, we berate ourselves and our actions, even as we lovingly nurture our families—especially our kids—and everyone around us. If you are like me, you're willing to give everyone else a little slack, a good excuse, but not yourself. Our sense of inadequacy or hatred and our limiting beliefs and shame work 365 days per year, and they show up faithfully to whatever event we're at; they're always on call. We can access them faithfully. Even if I am in the best moment of my life, I can find a way to change how I think and do something to where I feel inadequate. We're so skilled. But if we don't acknowledge our own self-worth, how can we possibly love ourselves and in turn love others?

I learned this lesson from one of my favorite Stimulati, Jorja Rivero. Jorja is an ebullient, beautiful woman with sparkling blue eyes, a slight Spanish accent, and feathers woven into her long brown hair. She consistently has a huge smile. She radiates confidence, understanding, and love. I describe her here because although we are not lovers, she is my own closest vision of authentic love outside of my family.

I first agreed to meet her after she was recommended to me, and the moment I stepped into her office, I knew I was meant to work with her. Jorja is a licensed master social worker (LMSW) as well as a yoga and meditation teacher. She has a master's degree from New York University and postgraduate clinical training from the Gestalt Associates for Psychotherapy. Her range of knowledge helped me broaden my understanding of myself and the human condition.

Jorja taught me to recognize that I am more than a mind, a heart, and a body; I'm an energetic, spiritual system that is in constant evolution. Her therapy is called healing living, and it is based on the premise that healing is how we integrate our experiences in a new way so that we can move forward into our lives with more depth, more complexity, more understanding, and, hopefully, more humaneness.

Jorja believes that we choose to live from either the ability to love ourselves or the ability to think that we're not enough, unworthy, inadequate, or unlovable. Your choice will create experiences that determine the way you perceive your life and the way you interact in the world. The way you talk to yourself and treat yourself and the choices that you make all have a distinct impact on your mind and your body. Self-love is therefore a conscious choice that we need to support and learn to choose. Please, choose it now! Even if at first it doesn't feel or come naturally, practice making this choice by putting yourself first, gently and with care. Self-esteem is all about learning to wholeheartedly love yourself, and you cannot do that if your self-talk does the contrary. You cannot be effective with others or receive their goodness when you cannot see, feel, or receive your own.

In Jorja's own words,

We are not aware of the amount of effort it requires to make a healthy choice until we start trying to make it. Hating ourselves also requires tremendous effort, one that we no longer experience as effort because we are so skilled at it. In order to love ourselves, we have to look at the areas of our lives that we typically don't want to examine. This is difficult, because we are inherently attracted to practices that offer a formula and a promise of some goal attainment versus learning to be in the ever-changing process of becoming, living, and healing.

For many of us, that dark, unexplored corner is the way we treat ourselves. As humans we all carry some stress due to the fact that we know we're dying and living at the same time. Now add to that our personal histories and circumstances, as well as the fact that we hate most of our needs, especially our inherent need for love, connection, and tenderness. We have a strong tendency to equate our needs with being needy, and we have great disgust toward our needs. We hate that we can't be perfect in the ways we demand we should be. These and other conflicts live inside of us, often as unfinished situations or energy loops that pull us back to the worst of our memories until we develop more awareness around those habitual patterns. In this way, our needs are a wise tool we ought to befriend.

Within ourselves, we are a multitude of beings and experiences. I believe we don't stop being 3 years old, 10 years old, 14 years old: All the ages we've been are still inside of us. We co-create our existence with those old and new parts of us. However, we find skillful ways to cover up painful memories, devising strategies for not feeling our old wounds. A lot of us have stopped feeling because we often confuse thinking with feeling, which it is not.

In order to live better, we have to make the continual choice to feel the impact of our last choice or the places where we had no choice. The more empathy we can give ourselves, the more we can feel the impact of our pain and disappointments and the more we can learn to love what we've had to endure.

For example, when I tell myself that I suck, and I feel the impact of that statement, my heart sinks, my sexual organs and drive for life shrivel, and I feel like disappearing. But after sitting with those feelings a bit, I can then begin to access my desire to choose a better way of being with myself.

Even if those feelings were linked to a past experience and you then decided how you deserved to feel, you can still change the ways that you respond to those feelings and to yourself. In order to change, you have to feel! Feel the moments when you had no choice and the moments when you then agreed to have no choice.

Understanding that you tried to protect yourself by hating your needs and feelings is important. It was a mechanism that you probably developed to survive an environment that couldn't meet your uniqueness and needs for love, connection, and attention. Healing redirects and unleashes the stuck life force that stops you from self-loving.

Some of our most negative patterns can and will get triggered, and when that happens, it's not a choice. We all have some level of post-traumatic stress. No matter who you are, where you've been, and what you've lived, you probably did not receive enough reassurance, empathy, and support to build a cohesive inner landscape. It is hard to admit, but we all have one or more areas in which we are shaky, struggling, or feel inadequate and unsuccessful. Our shakiness and insecurities will come about for different reasons. The nervous system might begin reacting to something in our past, and that's not a choice. But with work and effort, we can learn to respond to these triggers in a different, healthier way. New choices will stick only when we have to go into the mud of our existence and look at what's painful, what's not integrated, what is in conflict, what was traumatizing, what hurts. Maybe we weren't told how lovable we are or it wasn't reinforced enough.

Harnessing these memories creates a foundation of a new inner dialogue. This time you can choose to be more loving to yourself. Then you can go deep into yourself and look at the places that may need your well-deserved attention and healing, some reconnecting, a new wish, some restoring, or some cleaning up. This is what we do continually as we heal and live. Healing and loving yourself are an ongoing practice. You're never done knowing yourself. It's a courageous act to learn to love life with all the horrible things that happen to good people. Accepting where we are leads to an understanding that life is constantly changing and so are we, and that's more than okay; it is actually an opportunity. Self-love is part of living and healing, and healing is living. I don't simply forgive once and I'm finished, just as I don't live through something once and then I'm finished. Those impossible beliefs are a cruel setup that unleashes feelings such as failure. Part of living successfully and feeling like we're evolving is understanding that we move back, we move forward, and we stay still. In that process of going back, forward, being stuck, and standing again, we never know what event we're going to encounter that is going to completely retrigger a place in us that either we know well or haven't even touched.

Through practicing, we can teach ourselves to slow down and watch how certain choices trigger old feelings. Then we can choose something different. You might have to remind yourself six times per day that you're lovable, especially if other stuff is getting triggered, and each time you undo another knot of that old pattern or inner argument. The more we practice loving ourselves, the easier it becomes.

I learned that when you are living with chronic illness or some other suffering, you're living with your healthy self as well as your unhealthy

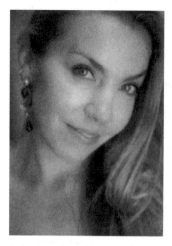
Jorja simply shines love.

self. A lot of our disease comes from not wanting to try something different and our insistence that the world is going to be the way it was yesterday and a minute ago, instead of daring to see that there can be something new happening right now.

Many times, illness is not a choice. However, what we do with it is a constant choice. Let's say you have an illness that doesn't progress or one that keeps getting worse, no matter what you do. Even though I believe that we impact our immune system and our overall well-being with how we live, there is another aspect of life that is completely random. Sometimes we do all the right things and something still goes wrong. Sometimes things happen with no apparent reason at all, and we can't control that. Those realities coexist. Even if we have the best attitude and we're not harboring any identified self-hatred, we can still cultivate mindfulness and awareness around the way we're feeling and loving ourself. The more aware and responsible we become, the more resourceful we'll be when things happen in life—and they will—to try to repair them to the best of our abilities.

Jorja also taught me what she considers to be a radical view about the relationship between forgiveness and self-love. She defines forgiveness as *the moment when we stop doing to ourselves what was done to us*. I liked this definition, because you don't have to necessarily forgive the act—the violence, transgression, or cruelty—and healing can take place completely on your own terms, as an act of your freedom of choice without involving anyone else. The continual work to undo hurt by being with myself is forgiveness. And it's ongoing, like life.

STIMULATI EXPERIENCE #8:
OVERCOME RESENTMENTS

If you are nursing an old hurt, stuck on a distressing episode, or ruminating about the could've, should've, would'ves of your life, then you have unresolved feelings that need to be cleared in order to welcome self-love.

I created the following exercise based on the teachings of Emmet Fox, a leader in the New Thought movement of the early 20th century. Fox was a minister, author, healer, and mystic. His teachings encouraged individuals to develop their own creative power. Fox believed, as I do, that we can lift our consciousness above the level of our problems and resentments in order to resolve them.

This visualization will help you clear your resentments. This exercise takes less than 5 minutes to complete, and you can use it whenever you become aware of feelings of bitterness. You can even use it in the moment when an unpleasant situation is occurring.

First get yourself to a calm, comfortable mental place. Then create a clear picture in your mind of the person toward whom you feel resentment. If it's yourself or your own actions, you can bring that picture to mind as well.

Think about the role you may have played in the stressful scene and how you might reinterpret the event. Imagine how the situation might look from the other person's perspective or a complete outsider's perspective.

Next, picture good things happening to yourself or that person. Is he receiving love or attention? Be aware of your own reactions. It may be hard at first for you to imagine good things coming to that person or yourself, but try not to be critical of your reaction. Accept it for what it is, knowing that it will become easier with practice.

When you are finished, notice how much more relaxed and less resentful you feel. Carry this new understanding of self-acceptance with you throughout the rest of your day.

BRING FORTH YOUR HEALTHY SELF

I know talking about self-love can feel a little awkward, but that's the essence of what we're getting at here. Just the idea of self-love or that you deserve self-love may make you uncomfortable, even squishy. Oftentimes we feel uncomfortable saying something positive about ourselves because it feels strange. That's why self-love is so difficult. Yet there's no better way to convey the act of having appreciation and affection for who you are. Although it sounds New Agey or hokey, it's true. It is what it is.

Jorja led me through the following exercise that uncovered my negative self-talk so that I could reframe it to create self-love and worthiness. The exercise led to physical experiences in my body, and for the first time in a long while, I understood that I was worthy and lovable.

The exercise begins with asking yourself a question: *If we all have a healthy self and unhealthy self within us, even when we're ill, what can I do to bring out my healthy self? What ideas can I change to believe that my healthy self is in there? How do I have to grow to believe and feel that possibility?*

Take your time: These are big, expanding questions. Listen closely to your self-talk and learn to then recognize the sensations in your body. Imagine what these sensations are communicating. You'll be surprised how quickly you can access what your unhealthy self wants to say. You may know some of its responses by heart, such as *you're a fraud; you're too old or too sick; you're not good enough for that.* But try to imagine what your healthy self wants and needs to say to you—even if you can capture only a glimmer of a feeling. For example, when we dwell on our worries, we create a stress response that is pervasive throughout our system. Can you connect the moments in which you're feeling the most pain to thoughts you are having, memories you are reliving, or people you are dealing with? It's like the lovesickness I described at the beginning of the chapter.

The more you feel that impact, or the toxicity and self-torture you produce through your thoughts and your denial of love, the more you get inspired to reframe your own self-talk to that of love and healing. These moments of insight shift the body in such a way that you can clearly recognize their impact. Then the next time you are triggered, you can choose to do something different.

Our imagination is a powerful motivator that allows our feeling process, living process, and visionary process to create a different experience. Through repetition and choice we make our healthy self a touchstone—that is, we create a new inner support as we weaken the charge and power of our unhealthy self. Our unhealthy self is not bad, and it needs as much love and permission to be heard and felt as our healthy self. That's why it's important to spend time in the mud with the parts of us that are in pain and feel helpless and to learn to heal and love them. Once we get used to this divide, ironically, we can feel whole. Then accessing our healthy self will feel more natural, and our unhealthy self will allow us to feel better. Being whole means we can hold the fullness of life—the full range of our human experience. Learning that each moment is a new opportunity and choice is a taste of freedom. We are responsible for ourselves, and that is freedom.

Give yourself permission to be something different by answering any of the following questions:

- How do you know when you're feeling healthy?
- What are some qualities you associate with feeling healthy in your mind, your heart, and your body?

- What are some ways in which you can relate to the world from a healthy place?

- How does it feel when you are stuck, low, depressed, or have strong symptoms? How do you perceive yourself, the world, and your relationships when you feel this way?

- If you didn't have those symptoms, what would you be able to feel?

Choosing to focus on the openness, ease, expansion, freedom, space, care, and tenderness that exists in your body cultivates self-love. Acknowledging that you had a choice and you chose something different—even for a moment—is worth celebrating. You can feel the empowering freedom from your old limiting pattern and feel a little or big glimpse of hope. Now you have something to measure for the future: not only a new feeling to think about but also an actual directly felt experience in both your mind and your body. Once you embrace that you are free to choose this feeling, you'll give yourself permission to choose it again.

Your new motto can be *I love myself and give myself permission to choose this experience freely. I have the right to feel good. Through my choices I create a feeling of ease and do not have to be stuck in my disease.*

A daily practice that has worked for me is doing at least three things that remind me of my self-worth. You can choose anything you are good at and that brings you joy. I choose to spend time every day writing, exercising or mentoring, and playing with my son and puppy to feel self-love.

STIMULATI EXPERIENCE #10:
VISUALIZE SELF-LOVE

Regardless of whether or not there is a real cause for your illness besides an emotional hurt and a mental fixation, the lack of love for yourself can exacerbate any chronic illness. This exercise may alleviate your symptoms.

While I can't promise a full recovery, I can tell you that after my breakup, I went back to zero, and now, just a few months later, I'm back at nine. Each time I get over lovesickness or other disappointments, I rebound better. We're constantly changing. The body is constantly creating a homeostatic situation in which it's self-regulating. You're already a different person than you were at the beginning of this chapter.

One way to cultivate self-love is a brief visualization. Picture yourself when you were 8 years old. In my mind's eye, I see myself as an 8-year-old boy, the same age my son is now. Then I ask myself, *what would I specifically do for him to protect him and motivate him to be his best self and feel the most loved?* This visualization reminds me that the answers to these questions are the same things I deserve to do for myself now.

THE LESSON OF LOVING OTHERS

All too often, people with chronic illness or any type of suffering isolate themselves. However, once you begin to love yourself, you can move beyond that singular relationship to connect with others. When you see your worth, you will have more to give to others. You will want to go out and meet people. You can allow yourself to become more vulnerable and open to the possibilities of creating and maintaining loving relationships. And when you create strong connections with others, you will feel less alone, less isolated, and less depressed. As your mood lifts, you will become more engaged with caring for yourself.

This idea isn't wishful thinking. At Remedy Health, we engaged Princeton Survey Research Associates International (PSRAI) to help us figure out how people dealing with chronic illness achieve the best health outcomes. Together, we learned that when people are friendly and open, they are happier, and when people are feeling happier, they are more apt to do healthier activities.

One way to become happier and more fulfilled is to determine and live your purpose in life. On the road to that goal, we also know that people become fulfilled and inspired by interacting with others. Whether it's connecting online, reading or watching a story, or talking in person, people feel empowered through these interactions to take more healthy actions and live healthier.

We also know that on a biological level, when you bond with others, either through a loving relationship or even a deep friendship, you ignite the love-body connection. The brain releases serotonin, a calming chemical, and lowers the production of the stress hormone cortisol. When cortisol is lowered, you experience enhanced serenity and happiness, and you feel better. A second brain chemical called oxytocin is also released when you're happy and engaged with others. Oxytocin is in the dopamine family and provides an adrenaline-like rush and blocks pain. Known as the love hormone, oxytocin is released when you're thinking about your loved ones or people who inspire you. This is another demonstration of how strongly we can control our health and mood. When stressed, you release cortisol; when in love, you release oxytocin. You're not a victim of your emotions: You control them.

STIMULATI ROBERT WALDINGER:
THE SCIENCE OF PERSONAL CONNECTIONS

Robert Waldinger, MD, is a Harvard psychiatrist, psychoanalyst, and Zen priest. He is the current director of the Harvard Medical School Study of Adult Development, which is possibly the longest study of adult life. For 75 years, his team (and his predecessor's) has tracked the lives of 724 men. About 60 of the original men are still alive and participating in the study, and most recently, he added over 2,000 children of the original participants.

His research and his plain-language TED Talk inspired me to reach out beyond myself and create connections. He was able to quantify scientifically what many of us already suspected: Good relationships keep us happier and healthier.

Year after year, his team would connect with the survey participants and through many types of data collection found that people who are socially connected to family, friends, and community are happier, physically healthier, and live longer than people who are less well connected. What's more, the experience of loneliness is virtually toxic: People who are isolated are less happy and experience physical and mental health declines earlier. Close relationships buffer us from both mental and physical pain. In his study, the most happily partnered men reported that on the days when they had more physical pain, their mood stayed positive. But the people who were in unhappy relationships, or lacked relationships entirely, had their physical pain magnified by their emotional pain. Despite any physical issues, the men who are able to develop and maintain relationships, and consequently live the longest, are also the healthiest and the happiest. The combination of interaction, community, and connection is what seems to be making people healthier.[1]

The second important finding from his research is that like everything else in life, it's quality over quantity. It doesn't matter if you have 1 friend or 1,000, nor it is important whether or not you're in a committed romantic relationship. The most important factor that predicts better health outcomes is the quality of close relationships of all kinds. And of course, if you have a purpose in life.

You can view his talk at www.ted.com/talks/robert_waldinger_what _makes_a_good_life_lessons_from_the_longest_study_on_happiness.

Connecting Via MyCounterpane

One of my favorite mood-tracking tools is found at MyCounterpane .com. It is a resource that asks you to break your story into moments that you can share and connect with others. What I like about it is that it offers each participant a moment of reflection as well as an opportunity to share your story with others: You can both reflect and connect in a safe way.

As people tell their stories, they tag each entry with one of 11 emotions (happy, hopeful, determined, aware, stable, overwhelmed, guilty, angry, lonely, scared, and sad), a date, and a brief description of why they felt that way. They can also add a band of color that represents their mood or a photo and a caption, or they can record video. Participants can lay out their past—starting with a moment they feel is particularly auspicious—and then continue to document their story in real time. Other people can then follow each story and leave comments, making the entire experience a shared event.

Kate Milliken, my friend I introduced in Chapter 1, created MyCounterpane when she was first dealing with MS. She told me, "If I asked you to tell me your story of whatever you're dealing with that's overwhelming, you might not be able to express exactly how you feel. But if I asked you to tell me your story from the moment you knew something was wrong, via your emotional ups and downs, whether it's been 4 days or 40 years, people remember that story in an instant. MyCounterpane.com allows you to recreate your story, laying out all the moments of your journey. You can focus on the highs and the lows, the dark clouds and the silver linings. You can think back to the moment when the first positive came out of the negative."

Once you post your story, you can choose one of three ways to share your graph. It can be totally private: Your graph becomes a private journal and is not linked to the larger website. You can choose to tag your posts as *community*, which means anyone who registers on Kate's website can see these moments. These moments come up on an activity feed, like a Facebook feed. Or you can choose to make your content completely public, which means it's going to be searchable by Google. Kate has learned that 51 percent of her users tag their content *public*. People can find that one moment, and by doing so, not only get perspective on themselves but also have the opportunity to help somebody else. Kate has found that as soon as participants make their story completely public, they have more of a sense of contribution and purpose.

For example, in February 2016, Kate was contacted by an active online blogger named Heather Love Leffel. Heather has MS and had an idea to poll the MS community on Mycounterpane.com and ask people with MS one question: *What have you lost because of your MS?* After people posted their video responses, Heather produced a single video of them. One of the respondents was Tracey, a woman who is bedridden and wheelchair-bound, who commented, "I've lost everything, but I'll still keep fighting." When the video was posted on Facebook, it received 21,000 views and 102 comments within 5 hours, the majority of which were supportive and complimentary. When Tracey saw the video herself, she commented, "Thank you again! It has not been a good week and this touched me. So I think I'll hang on a little while longer."

IF CHRIS CAN EXPERIENCE
A LOVING RELATIONSHIP, SO CAN YOU!

One of Kate Milliken's favorite stories is about Chris Guzikowski, who also has MS. When Chris started to use MyCounterpane.com, he was very depressed. He started tracking his mood back to the moment he knew something was wrong with his body: He was taking a walk in the woods and kept slipping. He marked that moment as feeling *overwhelmed and scared*. On the website, he continued to record his feelings over time. He marked the dates when he could no longer work in an office and when his world got smaller and his friends drifted away. His historical data ended with a date almost 10 years after the onset of his illness. At this point, he was for the first time at a place of acceptance of his illness and realized that he had isolated himself from the world. He was finally ready to meet other people with MS, and he decided he would reach out to them online.

Over the next year, Chris's moods continually improved. He went from feeling angry to determined and eventually to happy. He lost 135 pounds in the first year and started attending online MS community meetings. When he connected with other people, everything changed for him. Online, he met other people who had similar circumstances, and as he did, his mood stabilized as *aware and determined*. He set new goals for himself that addressed both his physical and mental health. When he felt more confident, Chris took the next step in reaching out and found an MS support group that met just 5 miles from his home. At the same time, he noticed a photo of a woman named Donna on another MS website, and they started an online conversation. He felt supported by the community to reach out to Donna and ultimately realized she was his soul mate.

Chris's entry from Valentine's Day 2015 best describes how important other people are to your health. He wrote, "This Valentine's Day was different from others. Before I was lonely and sad, but this year I was lonely and hopeful. I realized my previous goals were all about me . . . My new dream of happiness will involve someone else to accomplish my goals with . . ."

Chris continued taking better care of himself. Over the next 6 months, he consistently tracked his mood as both happy and hopeful. He eventually met Donna in person and, soon after, proposed to her.

In December 2015 the couple got married and, of course, posted it on the MyCounterpane website.

CONNECT TO PEOPLE WITH LOVE

Part of connecting to others is being an active listener. People who connect with others by listening to their story generate more hope for themselves by modeling their actions after others' successes. This is one of the main premises of Remedy Health, where we've studied the responses of our clients and tracked their health experiences. This is the reason why stories matter.

You can connect with friends, family, or even acquaintances you see in your town. Take an interest in them and listen carefully to their stories. Here's how you can start.

1. Create a list of five people you already know—your inner circle— who you want to connect with authentically and evaluate your relationships with each of them.

2. Then call and reconnect with your inner circle. Listen carefully to the other person's story. Curiosity is pretty safe: It's easier to find out more about other people than to tell your story. However, you have to be authentically curious: If you don't want to know the answer to the question, find another question to ask. People will know when you aren't interested in what they have to say.

   Here are some of my favorite conversation starters. They all allow the people you are speaking with to relive a positive feeling, which will open them up to telling more stories. Pose the question and then shut up and listen. Even if you want to interject, like when you know something about their story or could add to their story, don't. You don't have to fill an empty space in the conversation: Your silence allows others to tell more of their story.

- "I've always been curious about your life; would you be comfortable telling me more?"

- "I was impressed when a certain event happened. How did you feel about it?"

- Or create a question of your own, based on information you have about that person. It could be about their job, their family, their kids, or their pets—whatever interests you about them.

3. Get outside of your inner-core family and friends and connect with someone new. You run into so many people every day. Conversations like these can open you up to the possibility of meeting new people.

THOUGHT IGNITER

There is no difficulty that enough love will not conquer, no disease that enough love will not heal; no door that enough love will not open; no gulf that enough love will not bridge; no wall that enough love will not throw down; no sin that enough love will not redeem . . . it makes no difference how deeply seated may be the trouble; how hopeless the outlook; how muddled the tangle; how great the mistake. A sufficient realization of love will dissolve it all. If only you could love enough you would be the happiest and most powerful being in the world.

—Emmet Fox

CHAPTER 5

SURROUNDING YOURSELF WITH AWESOME STORIES THAT HEAL AND INSPIRE

THOUGHT IGNITER:

How can you give yourself permission to hope for more?

Hope is the spark that allows us to envision our future full of possibilities. It's the desire that encourages us to dream for something more than we have now. Without hope, we can't dream, and without dreams, we can't progress and evolve. Sometimes the stories we surround ourselves with sabotage our hopes and dreams. Is your inner circle filled with people who are positively supporting your dreams, or are they squashing your hope and bolstering doubt?

How do you take your hopes and dreams and make them real? How do you get that spark to ignite? In this chapter you will learn how to use your hopes and dreams as the catalyst to disrupt illness and struggle, eliminate fear, and remove yourself from negative influences.

BOO!

Let's face it, hope is a risky business and can be damn scary. In order to create any kind of change, you need to start with a vision, a hope. Yet sometimes, just having that hope can be scary. You may set your sights on a large goal or a big chance, and you may be afraid that you'll be let down—or even devastated—when it doesn't come together exactly as you planned or doesn't happen at all. All of a sudden, the What-if questions you ask yourself become a minefield, and even the most positive, uplifting hopes can leave you paralyzed in fear of failure or loss. When you're in survival mode, the safer route is not to have hope at all.

However, if you don't allow yourself to have hope, then you'll never get to where you want to be. And if you don't try to actualize your hopes, you can't be stronger, better, and bolder. As you become bolder, start to step outside of your comfort zone to achieve better health or a transformation and start to take the necessary actions to help you fulfill your dreams. Inevitably you're going to experience setbacks. When you are trying new things, not all of them are going to work exactly as you envision. Just because you didn't get exactly what you hoped for doesn't mean you failed. It means you got new insights and information on how to move forward more successfully, taking a slightly different path.

I learned this lesson a few years into my illness. I had already started the aggressive intravenous treatment regimen with Dr. Donta. Part of the protocol was to get an MRI every 6 months to see if the lesions on my spine were changing. One day I went to get the usual checkup MRI, and the lesions on my spinal cord didn't show up. There was nothing!

The MRI was clean! I remember I felt excitement like Christmas morning with a good dose of sigh-inducing relief.

I thought, *oh my God. It's over. I'll be walking and running and happy and getting back to exactly the way I was before I was sick.* In that moment there was so much hope. I reflexively started making a plan in my head for what things would be like when I was physically and mentally healthy again. Even though my symptoms hadn't changed much and I wasn't overwhelmingly getting better, I was still hoping I would have a full recovery.

Then 6 months later, I went back to get another MRI, which this time showed that the lesions were indeed still there. Maybe I had moved my body during the last MRI and the picture was blurry, the contrast was off, or the lesions had shifted. The doctors called the phenomena *waxed and waned in size and shape.* Whatever it was, 6 months later the lesions were clearly back—or had never left in the first place. And my symptoms—well, nothing was getting better.

All the hope that had been building inside of me came crashing down in disappointment. I felt exasperated and, quite simply, sad. Everything that I had been hoping for during those 6 months in terms of my recovery didn't happen. It was such a crushing failure and a loss.

That day I was at home at my parents' house. This was during the time that I didn't show any emotion or vulnerability about anything to the outside world. I left the house in a huff and drove to an empty parking lot. I got out of the car, laid down on the pavement, and cried, really wept. When I came back to the house and my eyes were red, my father thought that I had been smoking pot.

I didn't say anything. I guess I had earned that reputation, and because I didn't show any vulnerability before, he never imagined that I would be actually crying. Remember, you can't hurt Superman.

For days after, my life consisted of sleeping and watching bad cable

TV. This is where the people around you come in. Despite a good dose of dysfunction, I have always had an excellent support network with my family. No matter what, my parents and my sisters have shown up for me and have always been a positive impact. So has my best friend since third grade, who has become a successful record producer. Luckily my inner circle is solid. After about 3 days, my father brought me a razor and some shaving cream, and with some humor about my becoming a lumberjack, got me out of bed, into the shower, and cleaned up. My mother cooked my favorite meal, and my sister talked about what awesome opportunities the future held.

I knew that I could give up and stay in bed hoping to die or I could keep living the best life I could while looking for ways to heal. My people helped spark me out of my depression. I adjusted my hope to focus on different goals. After that experience, I realized that there were going to be lots of ups and downs as I found my way through this illness, and I could not commit myself to having any specific treatment work out exactly the way I thought it would. But that doesn't mean that the treatments were never going to work out.

I gave up the desire to find a definitive diagnosis. My hope remains to be healthy, calm, and confident. And because of this, everything in my life has eventually worked out. I'm still walking with a limp. I don't have the exact physical ability I did when I was 22, but mentally and emotionally, I'm much stronger, and I have found my purpose. I hope to go to Panama in the near future to receive treatment with stem cells.

Anything is possible.

Maybe you cannot depend on your family to help you stay positive and ignite your hope when you need a spark. Perhaps your family is a reason you are suffering. Consider this: Pessimism, negativity, and toxic people are poison for your hopes and dreams. The healthiest and most successful people surround themselves with positive, passionate, and open people. Try to limit your exposure to the toxic and use your community to surround yourself with stories of positivity.

I focus on having my hopes and dreams work out rather than determining how they will work out. This takes a little bit of faith. But when you start to believe and focus on the fact that everything will work out and you will be in a great place, it simply does.

I believe that there is no such thing as failure. Failure is a label that we put on our disappointments. It's true, the test results came back and they were positive. There were still lesions on my spine. But those truths didn't point to a failure of the treatment; they just missed my expectations. In the moment, I felt failure, but if I look at my life in its entirety, things, even back then, were working out. The world, the universe, my life were working out in their own way. Today, because of the realization and awareness I have gained from examining my own story, responding to events, and changing my mindset, I have been able to readjust to live with the belief that my life always works out and failure is a way to show me the next right step. Awareness is a powerful agent of change.

WITHOUT RESILIENCY, HOPE IS, WELL . . . JUST HOPE

Resiliency is being able to bounce back from hurt or harm. It is the understanding that failure is merely a temporary obstacle, a learning opportunity that opens the doors to other possibilities. It's another experience. It's not the end of the world.

You are already more resilient than you may realize. Take a moment to think about the small instances that have troubled you over time. The day you were diagnosed, that fight with a loved one, that relationship that broke up, that job that didn't work out. These events created real emotional upheaval. But as you think about them, think about where you are right now.

The majority of the time, you recovered. That breakup? You recovered and found a new love or passion or confidant. That argument that was driving you mad? Either you're friendly with the person again or you've removed him from your life and don't have that stress anymore. That job you hated? Maybe you're still in it or maybe you decided to find another job. Either way, you have a way to pay the rent.

If you look back on your life, chances are that many of these small instances didn't work out as initially planned. But each one of those so-called failures created more resiliency. If those situations happened now, chances are that you would do them differently: You would adjust your plan. Now you have real evidence of what worked and what didn't. What's more, you would also have more emotional bandwidth to understand that you are going to make it through.

Resilience allows you to focus on the big picture without regret for what no longer exists. It's not particularly specific. I use it as a tool to push through, to give me strength. I don't dwell on all the little things that can go wrong. Resilience is not a constant emotion or act—you use it when needed—and mixed with vulnerability it makes you unstoppable, because you are helping yourself and allowing others to help you as well.

My experiences have taught me not to get caught up in the details. In some ways, the least resilient people are the ones who get what is commonly known as analysis paralysis. If you're constantly analyzing your life, you're going to create more details and more disappointments. Or perhaps it is based in fear. If you keep planning and analyzing, you never have to take the next step forward.

Don't get me wrong: I think being detail-oriented is a good thing. But in some senses a bird's-eye view of life creates resiliency. You're not looking for every tiny thing that could go wrong. And when something does go wrong, you can recover quickly, because you are not attached to the outcome of every detail.

If you are spending too much time on the details and find yourself not moving forward with the big picture, though, take a step back, be aware of it, and reassess. Again, the details are important, but don't let them stop you. Focusing on the big picture still requires awareness, but it gives you the license to let go a little.

To see if you are stuck in the mud of detail, ask yourself:

- Are you getting caught up on one issue at work or in your primary relationships?
- Have you read about every symptom of a possible condition you might have and find that once you know about them, you start experiencing them?
- Are you stressing about what you will eat on the third day of your next vacation for lunch?

STIMULATI EXPERIENCE #12:
ASK YOURSELF, "WHAT DO I WANT? WHAT DO I REALLY, REALLY WANT?"

You likely already know what your issues are.

When you chill out and admit it, you even know what the main obstacle in your life is. But do you know what you are hoping for? The objective of this exercise is to identify your big-picture goals and subconscious desires for your health and your life. I'm going to give you two ideas: The first is to start to figure out how to ignite your life. The second hope is to start to figure out your purpose in life.

This exercise gets you past overarching hopes of *I want to feel better, I want less pain,* or *I want to be healthy.* It helps you determine a more precise wish, such as *I want to be able to go on a trip and not worry about how I'm feeling, I want to wear a sleeveless shirt despite my psoriasis,* or *I want to* get out and see the world despite my paralysis. Whether it's *I hope I can live longer to see my grandchildren, I hope I will lose enough weight so I can be more active and play with my kids, I want to be less depressed so I can get out of bed and go to work, I want to be married,* or *I want a new job,* it doesn't matter. Your hopes are your hopes, and whatever they look or sound like, they are completely valid. What's more, they're achievable.

I first learned about this exercise as a piece of group work. It's an interactive exercise that requires two other people to stand in front of you and ask *what do you want?* over and over rapidly in a bold, loud voice. As the third person, you must answer them as quickly as they ask, without thinking—no analysis, just free-associative response. Just let it rip! It takes only 3 minutes to complete, and you may be quite surprised with the results.

This exercise can also be done on your own with free association writing. Write down on a piece of paper your secret desires in the broadest terms. Don't think about it, just start writing, quickly. Then try to get to the heart of what you really want by whittling down your hopes into more-specific desires.

Still not sure what you can hope for? Read on, friends, and you'll see that hope often comes from learning about the experiences of others.

MAKE A BIG-PICTURE STATEMENT

Or you can use my motto *Oh, what the fuck, do whatever it takes.* This declaration is another tool to create a resilient state and focus on the big picture. It's a motivator to say, *I'm going to keep going, whatever it takes. If this treatment didn't work, what the fuck—I'll try something else. I can manifest anything, because nothing can stop me.*

When the MRI showed that my spinal lesions were still there, I could have easily said to myself, *I was hoping the lesions on my spine went away, but they are back. That's it; I'm done. Nothing is working. I'm not going to look for a cure anymore. I'm not going to dream, I'm not going to hope: That pain is too much. I'm not going to see another doctor. I'm not going to go to another holistic healer. I'm not going to do my research. I'm going to try to make some money so I can support myself and whatever happens, happens. I don't need to feel any better than I do right now.*

That way of thinking is perfectly understandable, but to me, it is not acceptable. Again, that's survival-mode thinking, and that's something we have to disrupt. If we give in to this mindset, we will never ignite our lives with happiness, health, and meaning.

Commit to being resilient throughout your life. I am committed to having the best life possible. I'm committed to being better for my family, friends, and those I love. I'll do whatever it takes. For example, stem cell research from human umbilical cords has reached a point where I will try that, because even after 20 years, oh, what the fuck, I'll do whatever it takes.

Life is hard; we're all struggling. Some people find less struggle, some people find more struggle, but I can guarantee, not everything's going to be easy. The people who are experiencing life to the fullest and having the most success are the ones who have fully realized hopes and the grit and resilience to get through it. They don't get caught up in the minutiae of what they perceive as failure. When their dreams don't work out the way they thought, they don't shut down. They keep going. They're ready to put themselves out there again, knowing that it will be okay if they fail.

If you can be the person who says, *Oh, what the fuck, do whatever it takes,* and it doesn't work out the way you wanted it to and you learned from the experience, you'll be able to say, *Oh, what the fuck, do whatever it takes* again. Eventually it's going to end up working out. But if your first reaction is to say to yourself, *Oh, God, I can't do that again, because last time it failed,* then you didn't allow yourself to learn anything and you've blocked any opportunities that could come to you. The next time, I guarantee that you'll feel like a failure again. Worse, you're totally limiting your possibilities.

THE A-HA MOMENT THAT LED ME TO HOPE

A few years ago, I was feeling disconnected. New York City's the most wonderful place in the world, but you need to take breaks from it. I had been working hard on launching Remedy Health, but the company wasn't clicking yet. I was feeling like I needed to get some perspective and recharge and get out of a rut.

Because I was resilient, I went looking for another avenue that would open something for me so that I could go forward on a more positive path. If I had been committed to having the company work out the way that I had initially dreamed, then I would have kept pushing what we were doing, not made any changes, and given up and gone to work somewhere else or tried to start somewhere new. But I knew that it would work out. How—I wasn't completely sure.

So I went on a spiritual retreat in the Arizona desert. I had learned about it from some friends who were working in Tucson. It was called a soul journey. I wasn't sure exactly what would happen, but I knew I would get to work with horses, learn about Native American shamanistic energy healing, and have some cool experiences that were the complete opposite of what I was currently doing.

At first I spent a lot of time meditating and allowing myself space to think about what was next and how things could work out as well as to hope for what I really wanted. It allowed me to have a much more open mind about what I should do differently and how I should pivot and change and keep going instead of following the same route.

But it wasn't until I began connecting with the other people on the retreat that I noticed a strong change in the way I was feeling and thinking. The people on the trip were great, although I can also say that they were neither special nor unique. They were regular people living ordinary lives; yet despite their struggles, they were doing well. Over the course of a few days, we learned about one another by listening to one another's life stories, and I became overwhelmingly inspired.

It wasn't one inspiring story that shifted my thinking. Each person had a different story of how she had overcome illness, had a challenge in her family, or had done something incredible in business. Each one had achieved something great despite the odds. Some of the folks had been practicing yoga for a long time because they had been in a car accident and yoga had changed their body and their life. Some people were healing in one way or another. One woman had been through a divorce. Another person was in a great place and was on the retreat to reconnect with the earth and feel grounded.

I realized that everybody has a story and people are in different parts of their story. No matter where they were, their story became a great catalyst for me to get to the place of thinking, *if they can do it, so can I.* As I spent time in the desert and meditated in the sweat lodge, I realized that with these real stories, more than anything I was learning on a spiritual level what inspired me to be . . . better. Being with other people and being infused with the inspiration of personal stories, I felt more hopeful and ready to overcome the obstacles in my life. I was motivated to do what I had previously thought was too difficult. I knew I was ready to change. I was eating better. I was exercising more. I wasn't feeling like I had to force things.

I wanted to share what I learned with everyone at Remedy Health. I knew that the power of stories might be the key to motivating someone from having hope to doing something. It turned out that my idea wasn't a hard sell. Storytelling has been around forever. Cavemen were writing on walls to tell their stories. In our modern life, people need to connect in an authentic and safe way with others who are going through the same things. They can learn from their experiences and be inspired by what they've accomplished. I realized that was incredibly easy to do online.

Support groups often serve this function. My challenge was to marry the benefits of support groups with technology in order to create an emotional connection through storytelling for anybody to consume right in their own homes. We started with the Live Bold Live Now empowerment initiative. We would find people who were going through traumatic events that anyone could relate to, who had overcome and triumphed over their condition. We started with a number of stories that we created in a multimedia-documentary style on HealthCentral.com, and we created seemystory.io as the storytelling platform for people to create their own multimedia stories and then connect with others like them within a specific health-related community. It allows people with chronic conditions to engage, connect, and act to change their own story.

In a few short months, millions of people came to watch these stories. The comments and the feedback were clear: These stories were truly inspiring, and viewers were motivated to get to the same place with their own health. I felt truly inspired that we were doing something good, and personally, I felt like I got back in flow.

STIMULATI REMEDY HEALTH AND PRINCETON SURVEY RESEARCH ASSOCIATES INTERNATIONAL: QUANTIFYING HOPE

Next we decided to research what kind of impact sharing stories has on patients and caregivers with regard to their health. We knew from our success at the Health Central website that storytelling creates hope. The question was, how much?

We surveyed 4,500 people living with a chronic condition. Initially, we thought the research was a bust. The study proved that patients were engaged in self-limiting views of themselves that kept them in poor health without motivation. The overwhelming majority—84 percent—identified themselves as happy and healthy. You read that right: Chronically ill people identifying themselves as happy and healthy. My first thought was that something was wrong with the survey questions. If you're chronically ill and identifying yourself as such, it's oxymoronic to say you are healthy. Either we happened to get the most positive chronically ill people on the planet in one shot or we needed to look deeper. Then I realized that the respondents were in survival mode. They were in the same place I used to be, accepting their life the way it was and living without hope that it could be any better.

We decided to stimulate the respondents. We showed a group an inspirational documentary that highlighted how one person cracked their survival mode of living with chronic illness and went on to have a better daily living experience. This time, when the respondents saw that the bar of happiness could be higher than their current situation, they indicated that they felt inspired and hopeful and more likely to take healthier actions in the future. The data suggested that inspirational stories were a catalyst to break down their survival mode. Specifically, 72 percent of respondents became hopeful when presented with an inspirational stimulus, which then helped them embrace their condition and come to terms with the idea that they could do better. In addition, 43 percent reported that after watching the documentary, they were inspired to see their doctors and explore new treatments, and 84 percent of respondents took an action, which included:

- 51 percent started eating healthier or more nutritious foods
- 41 percent started exercising more regularly or intensely

- 25 percent reduced or better managed stress
- 22 percent went to their doctor for a regular checkup
- 22 percent got more sleep
- 19 percent got preventive screening tests like a colonoscopy or mammogram

In short, when hope was developed via storytelling, more healthy actions were taken and people began to actually change their own story. Those actions helped them define what was most fulfilling for them, which led them to explore their purpose in life, which as we know can make you stronger, better, and bolder. This is why I say that hope opens doors to possibilities.

Your first response might be *No way, Jim, not me. These other people weren't hopeful. They beat the odds because they are superhuman or there was some kind of miracle.* My answer is that everyone has the potential to heal.

STIMULATI EXPERIENCE #13:
MAKE CONNECTIONS THAT INSPIRE HOPE

You can ignite your feelings of hope by finding others' stories that inspire you. Building community by embracing others, forming relationships, and being around people who inspire you leads to greater purpose in life.

SELF-HELP ALERT: You have to unpack it. This means you have to do the work to expose the reasons that you may be feeling poorly based on what you are holding on to emotionally. The people who have defied the odds aren't special; they've done the work. By doing so, holding on to the hope that things will work out despite the odds, and living a purposeful life, you too can be stronger, better, and bolder.

An inspirational story about a celebrity or a fictional story that motivates can make for great entertainment, but in terms of affecting your health, it is not a replacement for a real story from a person whom you can relate to. When you hear a story about someone like you who has achieved success, you start to believe the same can be true for you.

Everybody has a story. Your goal is to have a conversation with people about their life and what they've overcome. The key here is to be bold and take your hope wherever you can get it.

- Start at Healthcentral.com, Seemystory.io, or Medium.com and review any of the dozens of stories that are highlighted. Don't worry, it's free. Comment on the ones that are meaningful to you.

- You may know someone who has a story of triumph. Interview him: If he's achieved amazing things, model your story after his success. If he can do it, so can you.

- Join a support group or community and interact with other people.

- One of my favorite places to go for my story fix is StoryCorps at storycorps.org. These are real stories from real people. Who knows, you might be inspired enough to record your own story.

ROB HILL CONQUERED MOUNT EVEREST, AND YOU CAN CONQUER YOURS

One of my favorite inspirational stories is about Rob Hill (you can see his video at immersive.healthcentral.com/ibd/d/LBLN/living-with-crohns/?ic=herothirds). Rob was diagnosed with Crohn's disease (a chronic autoimmune disease that affects the digestive tract) in his early twenties. When he first experienced what he calls the scary symptoms of excruciating pain, diarrhea, rectal bleeding, and vomiting, he went from his primary care doctor to a gastroenterologist to the emergency room in under 2 hours. While medications have kept his symptoms somewhat controlled, he will have Crohn's disease for the rest of his life.

Crohn's disease causes inflammation that wears away the digestive organs, particularly the intestines. A year and a half after his diagnosis, Rob's condition was only getting worse. He found himself in and out of the hospital with some frequency. He dwindled from a robust 185 pounds to a skeletal 105. At his weakest, he could barely make it up a set of stairs.

The disease took an emotional toll as well. He was embarrassed about his symptoms, about constantly needing to know the location of a bathroom. He also felt lonely, as if he were a spectator in his own life. His poor health forced him to quit his job as a woodworker, and during the first year, leaving the house became physically impossible.

His doctors recommended that he have an ostomy, a surgical procedure where he would be able to discharge bodily waste into a bag attached to his abdomen. The surgery removed his entire large intestine, and while it was a success, Crohn's can occur anywhere in the digestive tract. For Rob, that meant he would have to have the ostomy bag for his entire life and still have many of the symptoms of Crohn's disease. When he awoke from the surgery, he was beside himself with depression but eventually realized that he had to make a choice. He chose to continue to live.

A lifelong climber, Rob created new goals for himself. He decided to focus all of his energies on climbing. He forced himself to become more physically active, rebuilding his body by running in competitive races and climbing. He also realized his illness was taking an emotional toll, and he actively worked at gaining a better understanding of Crohn's as well as his self-esteem. He found community by talking with others who were in the same situation and found that he became less lonely and more hopeful when he learned that other people were dealing better with the same disease. That community helped him develop the strength he needed to move forward with his life. He also found his purpose: to help other people with Crohn's disease get over the fear of the illness. He wanted to talk about living with the ostomy and the disease on a global level. He came up with a plan: to climb the seven highest mountains on seven continents in order to publicize his message. He would be the first person with an ostomy bag to scale all seven peaks. It wasn't easy, and he had other near-death setbacks, but he succeeded.

It took 8 years for him to master the first six mountains. With those successful climbs behind him, he hoped to climb Everest. The first time, he failed. He had to be taken off the middle of the mountain. His body collapsed on him. Yet he didn't let go of his vision or his hope. One the second attempt, he took along other climbers with inflammatory bowel disease, including a 17-year-old boy, Clinton Shard. After spending a few days at base camp, Rob's team went back down the mountain as he continued to the top, where he successfully summited.

Now he has dedicated his life to helping others with this same illness realize their dreams and release shame. He's living in a world of abundance. He learned that you can become the story your mind creates: In his case, his story is one of a mountain climber, and now he is one of the best.

His lesson is clear: You do not have to be your disease. You can hope for more. If you focus on sitting on the couch, taking your pain meds, and creating a story of pain, then that's what you're going to do. Or you can find your purpose, climb your Mount Everest, and take along another person to show him how to live stronger, better, and bolder.

THOUGHT IGNITER

Without leaps of imagination, or dreaming,
we lose the excitement of possibilities.
Dreaming, after all, is a form of planning.

–GLORIA STEINEM

CHAPTER 6

MANIFESTING YOUR PURPOSE WITH A NEW STORY AND SOME BOLD GOALS

THOUGHT IGNITER:

It's hard to reach the sun when you are shooting for the moon.

When I snapped out of survival mode and regained hope, the wants and desires came flooding in. I started hatching ideas and creating a vision for what was possible for my future, but I needed the tools to turn those hopes and ideas into reality. I needed to actually take those hopes and create a plan to fulfill them.

I started by crafting a set of new stories, each built around my hopes or a core belief about myself. I'd use these stories to communicate my goals or my new vision of myself. And little by little, these stories began to help me achieve my goals.

We all have many stories. Some are funny, some are tragic, some hopeful. One of my favorites is about a shaman I met in New York City. At the time, I was willing to go down any path and try anything that might lead to a cure. I was full of curiosity and hope, and I wanted to see what the world had to offer beyond traditional medicine.

Through a friend of a friend, I was connected to a visiting Ecuadorian shaman. He was in New York City seeing patients for a short time, and, of course, I decided that meeting him was a must-have adventure. I got an appointment, and I was told to bring a pack of Marlboro Light cigarettes and a newspaper to my session. Yes, you read that right. Perhaps even stranger than the instructions was the fact that I didn't ask any additional questions.

I went to the appointment with a good friend. We arrived at an old, dirty building in the East Village, a walk-up (meaning no elevator: of course *my* shaman was on the fifth floor!). So I pulled myself up the stairs, relying heavily on my arms and the railing, as I typically did. However, this time the railing actually came loose and I nearly tumbled down the flight I had just labored up. Despite the debacle, I was still raring to go. When we finally arrived, we were introduced to the shaman, who was sitting in a dark room wearing a white robe. All I could make out was a standing lamp, a desk, a chair, and candles. The perimeter of the room was surrounded by shells and some bones—which I hoped were animal.

My heart raced with anticipation. The shaman didn't speak English, but there was an interpreter, who told me to take off my clothes, lie on a mat on the floor next to the chair, and hand over the newspaper and the Marlboro Lights. I asked reluctantly if I had to take *everything* off, suddenly feeling anxious and wishing I had asked more questions ahead of the session. Again, it was shockingly odd, but I complied and stripped down without another word, wondering *what's the worst that could happen?* After a nervous glance my friend was allowed in and sat in the chair next to me.

The shaman lit a big branch of what smelled like sage and without warning started chanting and aggressively hitting my back and my legs with it. I jumped with shock, and it was then that I became fully aware of what I had gotten myself into. I was in a sketchy part of town, in a shady building, naked on the floor with a person whom I had never met and could not communicate with and who was beating me with burning sage while smoking my Marlboro Lights. All I could do was laugh. I looked at my friend sitting wide-eyed in the chair next to me, and we became hysterical with laughter. I worried that my laughter was offensive to the shaman's work and tried to stop, but I couldn't: It made it worse. I was now convulsing, trying to hold in each onset of giggles—which the interpreter said was a true exorcism of negative energy. Perhaps it was.

Afterward I sat up in front of the shaman and was greeted by puffs of cigarette smoke in my face. When the ritual was over, he told me that if I were to visit him in his home, he would certainly be able to cure me. He then gave me a small necklace made out of yarn and wrapped me in the newspaper. I was told to wear the newspaper under my clothes and not to change the paper or shower for a full week.

I never did go to his home, but for the next couple of days I went to work as he'd prescribed, crinkling around the office with newspaper underneath my clothes, smelling like sage and cigarette smoke. I told the story to my disbelieving colleagues, who were clearly unsure how to react. I told the story mostly because I was so self-conscious that I had to explain the noise the newspaper made every time I moved, not to mention the smell. But I quickly realized that this experience made for a great story that had to be told.

The shaman became one of my Stimulati. I do not believe that he had any mystical power (though I believe in the healing power of energy and native ritual. I recently visited with John of God of Brazil and had an amazing experience), but as with anything in life, you find different levels of talent and the rest is up to your interpretation and the intention you set. What he did do was give me a chance to show some vulnerability and create a great story that was the perfect icebreaker to get me reconnected with people. It allowed me to take out some of the heaviness in my old story, and I learned that my life didn't have to be so dire all the time. I didn't have to be so sick all the time. I could lighten my load.

You're not one story. You have your overarching story, which is your new set of goals. And within that story there are chapters. Share whatever you want. The stories you share don't have to be *I am sick; I'm depressed; I'm too weak—don't ask me.* It could be *you're not going to believe what I just did to get well.*

As your hopes become goals, you'll start to live your life through these stories, and they'll become your core experiences. My story's core beliefs are that I see the potential in people and opportunities. I'm proactive. I do things. I'm not afraid. I'm calm and confident. I know things are going to work out in one way or another, so I will take a risk.

When I started to share my shaman story, it opened me up to find more vulnerability in myself, which opened up yet another door to better health. The key is to be aware of the stories we tell ourselves and others and to live within them to the best of our abilities. Your goals, and ultimately your purpose in life, will come from your story. The next step is to be clear about what you want and how you bring this new story to life.

SETTING BOLD GOALS

Even if your new story isn't real yet, you have to start talking as if it were. Mindset science teaches us that we have to first be bold enough to actually say what we want. This takes courage, because it's almost like dressing for success. If your old story was *I'm not feeling great; I can't exercise; I don't have time; I'm overweight because I'm sick;* you can say that your new story is *I'm stronger, better, and bolder, and I can do whatever I need to do.* If you desire to be in a romantic, loving relationship and you haven't been able to find one, it's quite possible that you're stuck in your old story of *once I get better, I'll be able to find the right person* or *the timing is wrong.* Ditch it. Trade it in. Say aloud your new story: *I am love, and I am well enough for love. I attract love because I love myself, and I am ready for a relationship right now.*

One way to start living your new story is by visualizing what your life will look and feel like when it happens. Just as an athlete visualizes finishing a race or winning a gold medal, you can start to make your dreams come true by mapping out a new experience. In your mind's eye, form a mental picture of what the ideal outcome looks like when you are living your new story. Fill in as many details as possible. How does it feel to you? If you have difficulty conjuring this image up, look in magazines or on the Internet for photos that inspire you.

By beginning to live my new story, even before it happened, I was dipping my toes into the water of a better life. As I shifted, I started to feel grateful, as if I already had accomplished my goals. When you feel like you already have something, you open yourself up for it to come. I learned that if I was bold enough to take that first step, I would be able not only to accomplish my goals but also to see the next challenge and ultimately find my purpose. I went from being Jim, the man who creates stuff for a company and deals with a health condition, to Jim, the man who overcame chronic illness and suffering and has the ability to help others do the same.

Base Your New Story on the Right Goals

Sometimes having a flood of new hope can be paralyzing. If you can visualize your new story, you can get overwhelmed by all the ideas and then stop making progress toward achieving your goals.

You need to create a singular vision that can be accomplished by expressing a set of goals that are clear enough so that you can get what you want. Then you can develop the action steps needed to meet those goals. Remember, it's one thing to have hope and do nothing about it: That creates anxiety, because it remains an unfulfilled dream. You don't want to be a dreamer. It's important that you don't sit around hoping and waiting for things to happen for you. You have to be proactive, persistent, and bold in the sense that you have to set goals, go out, and take the necessary steps so that things will actually happen for you.

STIMULATI DENISE SPATAFORA: YOUR PURPOSE IS DEFINED BY YOUR "NATURAL BORN GIFTS®"

Denise Spatafora is a life and business strategist who has worked with hundreds of leaders. She is an amazing motivator and helped me focus on which of my hopes and desires to pursue. I chose to work with her because she has a unique ability to understand people and see the truth in every situation. She helped me unlock my fearlessness so that I had more clarity about how I could accomplish my goals. Her holistic approach helped me brainstorm, strategizing my hopes into actions.

Initially, Denise and I were working together because I wanted help with my business goals. Ultimately, she helped me put my new personal story into action, including becoming the person I envisioned and creating the relationships I was looking for.

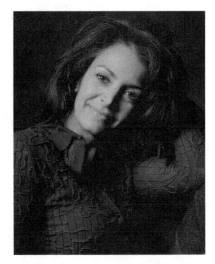

Denise, the master of getting clear.

Denise taught me that having goals is not just about knowing what you want. You will be pursuing the right goals—the ones that will help you find your purpose in life—when they are aligned with what she calls your "natural born gifts." Your gifts are the essence of who you are. Your gifts come across so naturally that you might not even acknowledge them as gifts. They are not your strengths, accomplishments, or learned behaviors. They are felt by others in the impression you leave behind and even the way you make them feel. They are your own unique stamp.

Denise told me,

People get confused and embarrassed when they try to figure out a few of their gifts. They even become uncomfortable, because it almost feels like bragging—saying too much about yourself. It might even feel overwhelming to acknowledge that this is the type of person that you are. But when you think about it, having that reaction is funny, because it is already who you are. It is already what people experience when they're with you, whether they verbally express it or not. In order to figure out your goals, you need to first peel back and identify two or three of your gifts. For example, my gift is that I'm a truth radar. I can see the truth in a second. I don't know why I have this gift, but I do. It's been like that my whole life. When people experience me, they'll say something like, 'Oh, wow. You're so refreshingly honest.' They'll say things like this, but what they're experiencing is the essence of who I am. I'm grateful to have this gift and have learned to use it in the work I do and in the relationships I have.

Denise helped me put my gifts into words. One of my gifts is optimism; I can also make people feel calm and comfortable in any situation. That's because I understand intuitively how most people are feeling in the moment. Denise refers to this as emotional intelligence.

There are times when no matter how hard we try, we can't silence the inner voice and we can't see or feel our gifts. It's not just you; this happens all the time and to all of us. We are all suffering. Welcome to being human. But if you are in such a dark place, you might need to get help before you can accept your gifts. Lift your burden by being compassionate and gentle with yourself, and get some help. Ask friends for recommendations and go online to find a therapist who is perfect for you.

Creating a Vision Board

You can figure out your gifts by trying to put your feelings into visual form. One technique I like to use to do this is creating a vision board, a tool to help clarify a specific life goal. It can be any kind of poster or drawing that represents whatever you want to be, do, or have in your life. Pick images from magazines or on the Internet that either convey a feeling or look like what your gifts represent. This may give you more access to finding the right words to name the gifts and allow yourself to trust that you own them. A vision board keeps you focused on who you want to be or what you really want and helps you achieve that desire. Say you believe that one of your gifts is connecting with people and inspiring others through your story, and you would like to be a storyteller or a public speaker. You would collect pictures for your vision board of people who are already doing that, such as Tony Robbins or Gabrielle Bernstein.

Put your vision board where you can see it upon waking up in the morning. When you get up, study your board, and visualize yourself already achieving your goals and desires. What do they look like? Feel like? Sound like?

Try to foster an attitude of gratefulness for what you already have, and say "thank you" for all the good things to come.

You can then set a strong, empowering intention for the day. Perhaps set an intention that says, *Today I will be my own best friend and not be judgmental towards myself*, or, *Today I will support myself by letting go of fear and focusing on my goals and desires*, or simply, *Today I am grateful for everything I have.*

By expressing gratitude and visualizing yourself achieving your goals and desires, you will be living in abundance, without the fear of not having enough, and with this, the Universe (and your mind) will provide.

Another way to identify your "natural born gifts" is to ask the people who know you best to describe your essence and find the similarities in their statements. Just by interviewing people, you're going to feel better, because you're relating and connecting. Make sure you listen to the positive feedback carefully, and try to silence the inner voice that might instruct you not to believe what you are hearing. This feedback will give you more access to the truth about your gifts, so you can see how much you are using and expressing these "natural born gifts."

Once you identify your gifts, you can begin to imagine what your life would be like if you started to align your goals with them. If you were using these gifts fully, what would you be doing and what would your lifestyle look like; what would be possible? How would you want to feel, mentally and physically? What abilities would you want to have? Your goals will align with those feelings. There isn't a right or wrong answer when it comes to your goals, as long as they are consistent with your gifts. For example, knowing that I am intuitive and optimistic, I learned that I could use those gifts to help others dealing with chronic illness overcome obstacles, as I did, which then became my purpose and the cornerstone of this book.

Denise believes,

> When you use your gifts to create the lifestyle you want, you will experience freedom. If your goals were created from using these gifts fully, you would experience your definition of freedom. Freedom is subjective, and just like your gifts, your experience of freedom would be all your own.
>
> If you are tapping into who you naturally are, then your goals will be consistent. It's your destiny. The next question is, what does that look like for you? For me, a truth radar could be a lawyer, or it could be an actor. I could use my gift in any way I wanted. As I create the next evolution of my business and my work, I use my gifts as a guide.
>
> You will begin to see your purpose when your gifts are being used in the most positive light. You know when your gifts and your lifestyle are aligned because there's ease. That doesn't mean that there will never be struggle. There are always obstacles. There is always hard work. You have to persevere and be resilient. But emotionally, you will feel it flow.

Once your gifts are aligned with your goals, you can start to create a plan, even a road map, for success. An effective plan is based on clear goals with milestones and committed actions. First set dates for when you believe you can accomplish these action steps. Then work backward and set two milestones between when you would begin the action and when you could reach your goal. These milestones should be 90 days apart. Working backwards, divide the next 90 days with midway goals between these two milestones. Decide what actions you need to take to ensure you hit the first midway goal. If you determine at the outset that you will not hit those mid-milestone goals, adjust your actions until you can envision movement and tangible results. Being aware of the effectiveness of your actions and using the two milestones as benchmarks will ensure you attain your final goals at the end of the period you have created. Be realistic about these goals without making them too small or so grand that you know they are unattainable

Let's say that your goal at the end of 90 days is to feel more vital and have more energy for travel, athletics, or whatever it is that you hope for. You want to run a marathon in the future—anything is possible! You'll have to set up clear expectations and a reasonable time frame. For example, the first milestone for the first 30 days could be to get out of your house each day and walk, building up your stamina in 10-minute intervals.

Then ask yourself, *what is my "natural born gift" that will allow me to reach this goal?* Refer back to the personality traits test in Chapter 1. Which of your personality traits can you call upon to help you reach this goal?

Then ask yourself, *what actions would ensure that I meet this milestone and eventually the goal of running a marathon?* You may have to plan your day more carefully or find someone to walk with.

After 30 days, you might notice that there starts to be a sense of ease in your walking. But if there isn't or you're finding that you're not making time for walking, then you have to reassess your action plan. That's where curiosity combined with resiliency comes in: What can you tweak to get the results you want? Are you taking responsibility and walking every day? Are you in pain? Do you have the right walking shoes and comfortable outfits? Modify your actions until you start to see results.

Set a second midway milestone for 60 days from your start date. At this point you could add lifting weights to build strength, push-ups, or flexibility activities like yoga. It's totally up to you to design your actions to whatever you think will make the difference and bring about positive change.

If your goals feel insurmountable, reexamine them. Figure out how you got to where you are in the first place. This kind of introspection is hard, and you have to be willing to dive into that. However, I can tell you that the work comes with rewards. You've heard others say about some part of their life, *I was down and out, but it was a blessing.* Be curious to discover why your obstacles might be a blessing. As you try different actions, what are you learning about yourself from them? Be willing to investigate.

In Denise's words, "Resiliency is sometimes forcing yourself or driving or pushing. That takes a lot of energy. But if it's mixed with curiosity, there's a lightness about it. If the action steps don't work, you try a different strategy. It's almost like you're a scientist experimenting with a breakthrough for yourself. You might think, 'Okay, look. I'm not going to get mad or frustrated, but I need to figure out what's not working, and why.' Do not invalidate yourself by changing your actions too quickly: Don't give up until you've reached your milestone date. Even small change is positive movement."

Then set the next milestone for 90 days from your start date. This time you might want to continue walking and start looking at your food choices. After 90 days, you may not have dropped 50 pounds (that would have been an unrealistic goal); however, if you continue to stay on point, you'll see improvement. More importantly, you're building a stronger lifestyle foundation that can help you sustain better health. What's more, by the end of 90 days, you very may well have fulfilled your first goal.

However, if you find that after 90 days you still have not met your first goal, it's time to reevaluate and see how much you want the goal. See if it's aligned with your gifts. And see if you want the goal for the right reasons. For example, if you thought your goal was to be more vital but deep down you were fixating on weight loss, you might not achieve your goal. This is why in most cases, diets don't work. You're going to give up, because losing weight to fit into your clothes is not a high-enough purpose. Instead, focus on your bigger goal of becoming more vital and you'll see that by creating more action steps that are aligned with your lifestyle and your gifts, the weight will come off. The weight is a natural outcome to being consistent. The results are the way to measure if the actions you're taking are the right ones. If you're not using your gifts, your results are probably slowed down, stopped, and/or stuck.

What's more, as you meet your goals by following your action plan, you will have greater clarity and start to see your purpose. That's a sign that you are on point and your ideas may already be starting to come together. Once you figure out what your gifts are, you realize what you are innately best at and how you can contribute your energy to others.

The goals and action steps are a critical process to help you get to your purpose. Goals start with understanding your gifts. Once I understood that I can make people comfortable and at ease, I realized that they can be in flow themselves and have better thoughts and ideas and identify their potential. That's my gift, but it also leads to my purpose, which is creating businesses that allow people to have better health, to connect people with experts, and to write a book that can help others identify their own purpose and their struggle a little bit.

I am constantly working toward several lifestyle goals. The first is to have flexibility in my schedule, to enable me to live where I want and work with whom I want, so that ultimately I can use my purpose to reach a mass audience. I also want to be able to do all of that physically, without pain: I want to travel with ease, without worrying about where the bathrooms are located, how I'm going to get through the airport, and how I'm going to get to the hotel. The action steps I took included getting a coach (thank you, Denise!) and figuring out the milestones I needed to create to meet my physical goals. In order for me to live more flexibly, I needed to lose weight. I needed to go to the gym every day.

Another action plan revolved around my purpose: How could I create the tools and information that could get to the most people? For example, Denise was the catalyst for me to write this book. She helped me discover my message: what I wanted to say and how I wanted to share the knowledge I had gained. Then we talked about what it would take to get a book published. Specifically, we put goals in place around getting a proposal finished, having the book selected by a publisher, and then writing the book.

The third action plan revolved around my personal life. I identified exactly what I wanted: a joyful, passionate, loving, and trusting romantic relationship. I also wanted to have a better relationship with my parents, and I wanted to commit to connecting with friends. I needed to remove negative relationships and focus more on what I needed and the people who were beneficial to me, not the folks whom I was seeing potential in or hoping I could change.

I'm happy to say that my goals worked out. I lost 40 pounds. I'm experiencing significantly less pain. I go to the gym quite often. My lifestyle is healthy. I eat healthy. I'm happier. I don't have destructive relationships. The book is written (hope you enjoy it!), and I have speaking engagements lined up where I can share my story and my message. Together we can reach your goals, too.

BE PATIENT WITH THE PROCESS

While my goals are working out, I'm the first to admit they have not been exactly as I imagined. And I'm still not finished. There have been many bumps in the road. I found myself in more than a few bad relationships. I lost money in business deals; I've had ups and down with my weight and pain. I needed to be patient and give myself time to conquer each obstacle. This particular journey has taught me that patience is as important as resiliency when it comes to creating the lifestyle you want. If you are focusing only on how quickly you can accomplish your committed actions, you may skip over the emotional growth that accompanies success. So as you work on your actions, ask yourself periodically, *how do I actually feel?*

Patience allows you to have compassion for yourself: It's integral for self-love. That's why I say that your goals will work out, just not always as you initially imagined. Again, this requires courage, resiliency, and curiosity. You already have the hope to get over your hurdle. It might not happen as quickly as you want, and that's okay. Give yourself the time for your goals to manifest, and be realistic and aware when your attempts at patience might be turning into procrastination, false hope, or an attachment to a particular outcome. Be prepared to find a new way around any obstacle you encounter.

> **SELF-HELP ALERT:** The journey itself becomes your new story, and you may be surprised where it takes you. With patience, you can expect additional benefits related to your goals that you could never have predicted. It could be a lightness, a clarity, or a sense of ease. You may find that you're now able to communicate better and have a deep impact on others.

CREATE GOALS AND A ROAD MAP

To keep all the pieces in place, create a road map that outlines your goals and a plan to achieve them. Setting firm goals, writing them down, and tracking your progress helps you to have a higher probability of achieving them. If you create an agreement with yourself, you'll be accountable to it, and it's more likely you'll reach these goals or see where you went awry.

Divide your goals into four main components: mental health, physical health, relationships, and contribution. For each category, identify where you want to be in the next 90 days. Quantify your committed actions as clearly as possible. Then every week, track your progress and see if you've achieved your goal or not.

I gave each goal an actual date for completion. You have to commit to your goals and your actions, but you can be flexible in how they work out. For each of the committed actions, write it in the most positive voice (i.e., *I will*), as if you're manifesting it. There's no room here for *I might be, I would like to be* statements. When you show conviction, you will make what you want happen. As you're reviewing your goals, you open yourself and your mind to accomplishing them. This is what allows you to create a new story, moving from *I'm single and alone* to *I will be in a joyful, passionate, and loving relationship soon.*

Here's a road map that I created for myself a few years ago. I would review this every day to make sure I was on track with my goals. There's a blank version in the back of the book for you to create your own.

My Road Map

Over the next 90 days, I will:

MENTAL HEALTH

Goal: Live calmly and confidently in a healthy and aware way.
Action:

1. I will meditate every morning for 15 minutes and go to the Kadampa Meditation Center once per week for a 2-hour class.

2. I will be present and observant in every face-to-face conversation I have.

PHYSICAL HEALTH

Goal: Become more physically fit so I can be more limber and have a less painful body.
Action:

1. I will swim 1,000 yards 5 days per week.

2. I will lift weights 2 days per week.

3. I will hire a stretching coach 1 day per week for a 30-minute session for a month and stretch on my own every afternoon.

RELATIONSHIPS

Goal: Have happy, open, and supportive relationships with friends and family.
Action:

1. I will visit my parents, have an open and honest conversation with them, and express my forgiveness and gratitude.

2. I will call my parents every Sunday for more than 20 minutes to create connection and love.

3. I will recommit to and create connected and loving relationships with friends by making calls and getting together with those I have lost touch with by making 10 calls and going to 2 events per week.

CONTRIBUTION

Goals: I will contribute to supporting others in the world without the fear of not having enough myself.
Action:

1. I will create a scholarship at the University of New Hampshire, my alma mater.

2. I will raise money for Project Sunshine and donate 10 hours to working with kids.

3. I will help five new entrepreneurs create their business plan and speak to potential investors.

4. I will write a book.

STIMULATI EXPERIENCE #15:
RETAKE THE PURPOSE IN LIFE TEST

Go back to Chapter 1 and retake the Purpose in Life Test after 60 days of working on your road map and see how your scores are changing. See where you were low in the test, and make goals to get what you want in order to increase your purpose in life. Setting and examining your goals will lead to clarity around your purpose.

BUILDING CONFIDENCE AS YOU TELL YOUR STORY: THE POWER OF CONNECTION

Whether you're an introvert or an extrovert, humans are social beings that need interpersonal relationships to survive and be happy. However, if you are struggling, you may find your circle getting smaller and smaller. You might rationalize this when you are in survival mode and say that you don't need people or that you are better off alone. This, my friend, is a false construct. It's a defense mechanism so you don't have to be vulnerable or feel the pain and sadness of your predicament. In fact, you are actually self-isolating when you say, *I don't need anyone; I'm good; I'm alone; you know, I've taken care of myself this long, I can continue to take care of myself.*

Recognize that you are building a new wall, a defense mechanism. You close down and actually stay in the same place or get worse, because we're inherently social people. And as social creatures, we are allowed to have both bad and good experiences and feelings.

In order to break down this wall, you need to tell one of your stories. Within Princeton Survey Research Associates International (PSRAI), we have found that when you share your story with others, you can more effectively change your own story and begin to heal. It's my hypothesis that once you have your goals and a vision regarding how you will achieve them, you will be more successful when you surround yourselves with others who can help. You can't accomplish your goals alone. The key is connection. By sharing your story, you realize that other people will become inspired, and because you know that you've inspired them, you find significance and purpose in life. In our study, the people who have triumphed and told their stories have developed an enhanced sense of well-being. Their contribution makes them feel a sense of obligation to live up to being a role model, and because of this, they take better care of themselves.

Become an Authentic Storyteller

There are two different kinds of stories. The first are the stories that we tell ourselves every day. For example, one of my stories is that I'm calm, confident, and I know that everything will work out for me one way or another. That's the story of how I am, what I believe, and who I am.

When I tell a broader story of my experiences, such as the story of the shaman, it reflects the primary story. You can tell by reading about my trip to the shaman that I wasn't writing it from a place of fear. I tried the experience, I moved on, and in the end, it worked out because it made me feel lighter and vulnerable. So in this instance, I took my basic core-belief story and turned it into an experiential story that people can connect with me about. I can use it anytime to motivate others or contribute in some way.

Everything we say and do is basically a story, and our core belief, that core story, is what we want to start to experience as a through line in every story we tell. Look at the stories you tell and see the nuances of the words and the way that you frame them, then change them to meet your goals and gifts. Start your story by anchoring it with what you've identified as your gifts. For example, if your core beliefs are *I'm not good enough, I'm going to fail*, and *I can't do that*, your stories are oftentimes negative. In regard to the shaman story, a negative version would have sounded like *my friend forced me to go, and reluctantly I went. When the railing broke off, I took it as a sign that the appointment was not going to go well.*

The stories then become examples of how you're living your life. I've identified that one of my core gifts is that I can make people feel comfortable because I'm not nervous and that I know everything will work out one way or another. When I tell a story, it's like that, so it expresses my core gifts without my saying, *this is my core gift*. You want to be socially and emotionally aware. You don't want to go up to someone and tell them a story about how awesome your gifts are. Instead, think of your story as a tool to create your goals through your authentic, every-day conversation.

To become an authentic storyteller, you have to speak from the heart, be honest, and relate to your audience with vulnerability. You have to be authentic: You are not necessarily telling a story to impress or entertain; you're telling it from your truth. Include real examples of what happened and how you feel, and try to relate to how others will feel when they hear your story.

Telling a great story takes practice and refinement. It's important that your story has a start and an end and is descriptive. Pick a point in time that means a lot to you, one that you're aware of how it could affect someone else. It can start with when you were diagnosed or your toughest moment or when you turned the corner and had a real change for the better. It could be a triumph story. It could be a story about the shock of when you first learned that you were sick, or it could be a struggle story about how you made it through the toughest times. Each story is inspirational in its own right and allows you to release a burden off your chest as well as connect with others who may have felt the same way. Remember, connecting with others, and letting them know that they are not alone, allows you to contribute to the world and feel significant.

Once you're ready with your story, share it! You can start to share a story by telling your family and friends. As you become more comfortable with it, widen your audience. Connect with passion to what you're saying. Try to relive the story as you're telling it. Make eye contact, move your body, and modulate your tone.

Or post it on social media. Promote it on Twitter. A 2016 study published by Facebook and Carnegie Mellon University in the *Journal of Computer-Mediated Communication* found that personalized comments or posts from strong Facebook connections were associated with improvements in well-being, equivalent to having a wedding or a baby.[1] That's an encouraging form of connection!

We talked in earlier chapters about how social media has been destructive, but there is a positive side to it as well. On one hand, it allows you to connect with your circle not only on your time but also on others'. You're defining your circle and you're connecting with it as often as you want, and it helps you share and contribute more easily. However, when you start to base your significance on the responses of others, then the value gets distorted. A forum like www.seemystory.io or medium.com is a more supportive social media experience, because it offers storytelling tools that help you talk about struggle without connecting to specific individuals. Oftentimes Facebook is not the most appropriate place for this type of storytelling.

STIMULATI EXPERIENCE #16:
USE STORYTELLING TOOLS

The storytelling tool we've created at Remedy Health allows you to include pictures, video, and audio to get your story across in the best way possible. You just have to be authentic and answer the questions honestly. Go to www.seemystory.io or medium.com to start crafting a new, bold story.

RAINA SHARED HER STORY
AND BOLDLY OVERCAME ADDICTION

Raina Lowell has battled with anxiety since she was a child. Yet her entire world changed when she took her first prescription painkiller. When Raina was 30, a doctor prescribed opiates to help address chronic back pain. When the Vicodin hit her system, she felt like she could breathe for the first time in her life. The pressure, loneliness, and fear were instantly lifted every time she took a tiny pill. So she continued taking the medication in private. She didn't talk about it with anyone, including her husband. She went to great lengths to fund her habit. She stole money from her business, stole from friends' homes, and wrote bad checks. When her marriage collapsed, she used all of her welfare and child support to buy drugs. Her close friends drifted away, and her children suffered from neglect. She lost her ability to connect with the real world.

Raina found a rehab facility and for the first time met other addicts. But instead of healing fully, she learned new tricks that took her deeper into her addiction. Soon Raina became a crack addict and a heroin user. Her sisters stopped speaking to her, and her ex-husband wanted to take her children away. Even her mother, who had been her ally, could not recognize the woman she had become.

When she hit bottom, she was living in an unheated house with her children during a Vermont winter. The conditions of the house were unlivable. She stole firewood from friends and started to burn her own furniture, because every dollar that she could find went to supporting her habit. Raina knew that her life didn't have to be this way, but she no longer had hope that it could ever improve. Life became too painful. She didn't want to live in the nightmare anymore. But her love for her children kept her going, and she made a promise to herself that she would try to get sober. If she didn't succeed, she had a plan to end her life.

Raina entered into a retreat for an entire year while her mother cared for her children. This time, she worked harder than ever, took every class that she could, and surrounded herself with people with similar goals. Today, Raina has been sober for more than 4 years. Sobriety gave her the opportunity to reinvent her story and become the person she always wanted to be instead of continuing to feel like she was not enough.

Slowly, Raina was able to put her life back together. She reunited with her children and started to work with other addicts. In 2014, Raina began to share her story, and she believes it was an integral part of her healing. She participated in a documentary called *The Hungry Heart*, a startling look at opiate addiction. She was the keynote speaker following the Vermont governor's state of the state address, where she shared her story with more than 300 people, who gave her a standing ovation. Raina believes that sharing her story keeps her journey present in her life and reminds her of how far she has come. She maintains her sobriety by actively participating in a 12-step program and attending AA meetings, and she shares her story with the entire world on her blog (howtoloveadrugaddict.blogspot.com). She also shares her story at Healthcentral.com (immersive.healthcentral.com/chronic-pain/d/LBLN /rlowell-living-with-addiction/?ic=caro). She now feels that she has come out of her experience a much stronger woman and a better person.

Raina's story shows me that once she realized that her gift was the way she could positively relate to other addicts, she was able to reach her goals, which were to re-create her family and reunite with her children. She used her story to contribute and become a respected advocate for people struggling with addiction.

EVERY STORY IS IMPORTANT

In this book, I've shared some of the most powerful, extreme stories I've come across. Raina's story, for example, is a big one about her life, where she experienced going all the way to the bottom and back up to a place where she's become an advocate for change. However, don't let these big stories intimidate you. There is no story too big or too small to share. Don't read someone's story and feel like yours is now insignificant. We all are struggling, and there's no struggle that's bigger or smaller than someone else's. So don't follow the rabbit hole of judgment or become afraid to tell your story. Everyone's story is significant because it reflects what you are feeling, and that is important.

Some of the best stories I've come across fall in the category of *to be continued.* Your story doesn't have to have an ending yet but rather a future vision. Most of us, myself included, are living in the middle of a story. And just because you know you're in the middle of it doesn't mean you don't have a story to share. For example, when I say that my story includes the goal that everything will work out for me, I'm not saying everything *has* worked out for me. I'm still in the middle of it. In fact, I'm 41 years old. I have another 41 years or more to work out the details of my story.

Your smallest story could turn you into a Stimulati for someone else. You know when you've become a Stimulati when you're living your story authentically and you can share and contribute your experiences in a way that ignites others' potential, hope, vision, and passion. Being a Stimulati comes with a feeling of empowerment for yourself as well. That is the contribution: It always gives back if you let it. You will feel as though you have meaning and purpose, and I promise it will make you feel stronger, better, and bolder.

THOUGHT IGNITER

Who will you be a Stimulati for?

CHAPTER 7

FINDING THE FORMULA FOR HEALING AND HEALTH

THOUGHT IGNITER:

What does it mean to live it and give it?

Connection + Worthiness leads to Contribution

Contribution leads to Purpose

Purpose leads to Significance

Significance leads to Healing

W hen I was in survival mode, I didn't feel worthy. I was performing work at a high capacity and often winning awards. But whenever there was too much attention on me, I felt like a fraud. I thought the awards were a farce, because I didn't believe I was valuable. In fact, most of the time I felt my work life was a sham, that I was fooling people. I would think *if people really knew me, they'd realized I'm not that good at this.*

The nagging doubts and the fear of being found out a fraud held me back from getting better. I didn't think I deserved to take care of myself. I stopped seeing new doctors, finding new treatments, exercising, or eating healthy food. And when I did break out of survival mode, after meeting so many Stimulati and working with them, I didn't see the connection between my gift and my purpose. For instance, I've wanted to write this exact book for many years, but then I would think *do I really have it figured out? Do I really have any value to give?* and I'd walk away from the computer, accomplishing nothing.

It wasn't until I actually started to share the story about my illness and my experiences that I realized I did have value and that I could significantly help others. When I started to do some public speaking and seminars, I could see how people were positively affected by my experiences. I could connect and ignite potential, hope, and passion, and this contributed to my feeling worthy.

YOUR BEST WEAPON AGAINST DOUBT

If ever I slip back into limiting beliefs such as *I hope I'm good enough*, I have to remind myself that feeling worthy is a choice that only I can make. I choose to be loving toward myself and to stop feeling guilty and shameful about my illness. I'm going to get better and I'm going to work on my mental attitude, because I'm worth that effort. I try to be aware of when I'm spiraling out of a place of abundance and into doubt. When I do spiral, I remind myself that I have the ability to love and therefore I am love, and love is always worthy. Sometimes ya gotta fake it till you make it, and the more you tell yourself this, the more you'll come to understand that it's the truth.

Another trick I use to take the pressure off myself is to focus on helping others. I remind myself how I help and positively affect people.

There's no greater proof of your worthiness than your ability to contribute to the world. That's why I think, *when in doubt, focus out.*

However, there's a huge difference between using your gifts to help others and being a people pleaser. A pleaser is a self-imposed denial trap: It's a trick to push aside the need to take care of yourself. That's not what I mean by *focus out.* A pleaser wants to make everybody else happy and comfortable all the time. Although it seems that pleasers are generous, their actions come from a place of having nothing. When you live to please others, you are not recognizing your self-worth and that you deserve help first. Instead, you're willing to bend, shape, and contort yourself and your beliefs to make the people in your life happy.

When it came to relationships, I was definitely a pleaser. It wasn't until I realized I could contribute just the way I was that I could put my needs first. I didn't have to please people all the time. There is power in doing what you want for yourself. Try it out, but don't be malicious. If someone asks you to do something and you don't want to or have something you would rather do, decline politely or firmly and say no, depending on what's appropriate at the time. See how you feel sticking up for yourself: I am willing to bet you'll feel pretty damn good.

SELF-HELP ALERT: Once you connect to others by listening and sharing stories, you'll begin to see how others are benefiting from having you in their lives. That's when you will come to understand your own self-worth. You may notice that you feel differently and perceive the world differently. You'll realize that you deserve to be happy and healthy. You deserve love in your life. You deserve to struggle less. You deserve to feel less anxiety and know that you're good enough. You're not a bad person. You have value. Your needs are important; taking care of yourself is important, because you have real gifts that you can contribute to the world. Give yourself permission to feel worthy. If you believe that you are worthy of health, you'll believe that you deserve it and will therefore be more apt to take the necessary steps toward becoming stronger, better, and bolder.

In the end, pleasing doesn't work, because you're constantly trying something new to affect someone else's happiness. It's inauthentic. You can try to change yourself to be funnier, more serious, or more competent, so you can make a parent, significant other, colleague, or boss happy. But what others see is a person willing to do anything to fill a void where self-worth and self-love should be. Help others, but remember, you have a backbone for a reason. Use it!

Pleasing behavior leads to codependency, an ultimately destructive relationship in which two people become so invested in each other that they can't function independently. Typically, one person requires help and the other becomes either his sole support system or his enabler. The classic codependent relationship is one between caregivers and the people they are supposed to be helping. You might have unknowingly developed a codependent relationship if you are sick and rely on someone to complete daily tasks. Or if you're constantly worrying about making other people happy, you might be creating a codependent relationship. When we are caring for someone with a chronic illness, it's quite common to stop taking care of ourselves, as we are 100 percent focused on the disabled son, the alcoholic husband, or the partner with lupus. It becomes easy to base our life around caring for that person. While we may be making the ill person more comfortable, better, and at ease, we are at the same time enabling that person to wallow in his suffering instead of giving him the tools that might lead to independence.

Surprisingly, many people living with chronic conditions also become codependent and find themselves taking care of others and neglecting their own health. Becoming a caregiver may seem contrary, because usually someone with a health issue gets a caregiver who then becomes codependent with him or her. Yet it is a common relationship to find yourself in when you are in survival mode. I'm guilty of this myself. In a previous romantic relationship, I was far more focused on the well-being of my girlfriend than taking care of myself.

Some of the telltale signs are if you don't have time to take care of yourself and you don't feel worthy enough to take care of yourself because someone else is suffering more. According to an article featured on Psychcentral.com, signs of codependent behavior include:

- Taking responsibility for someone else's actions
- Worrying or carrying the burden for others' problems
- Covering up to protect others from reaping the consequences of their poor choices
- Doing more than is required at your job or at home to earn approval
- Feeling obligated to do what others expect without consulting one's own needs
- Manipulating others' responses instead of accepting them at face value
- Being suspicious of receiving love or not feeling worthy of being loved
- Being in a relationship based on need, not out of mutual respect
- Trying to solve someone else's problems or trying to change someone
- Life being directed by external rather than internal cues (*should do* versus *want to do*)
- Enabling someone to take your time or resources without your consent
- Neglecting your own needs in the process of caring for someone who doesn't want to care for herself[1]

What's scary is that there is a real, albeit unhealthy, benefit to codependency. The caretaker feels needed, which is a wonderful feeling. However, you won't live at your best when you base your entire value and beliefs about your worth on this single emotion. And worse, when the caretaker's assistance is no longer needed, he crumbles, because he has not built up his own sense of self or self-love. Or he puts stumbling blocks in the way of the other's recovery in order to maintain his role as caretaker. Ouch.

If this sounds like you or someone you may be close to, it is important to practice the tools to develop your own sense of worth. Breaking this kind of relationship is going to be painful at first, but know that pain is temporary. You'll be able to get past it much more easily if you ignite a new passion and purpose.

Codependency is the antithesis of contribution. When I'm taking care of myself, I'm strong enough to help others. I'm coming from a place of healthiness and emotional strength. That's not to say you have to be perfect to focus out. Not at all. You don't have to be the healthiest or the wealthiest person to contribute. You simply have to come from a place where you're contributing to yourself first. If you don't, you're contributing from a place of need; you're giving with an expectation or a hopeless desire that you will be loved.

To break out of a codependent relationship, you have to put up real boundaries until you are strong enough to believe that you deserve to have your needs met. You need to fill your own proverbial gas tank before you can truly help anyone else.

STIMULATI EXPERIENCE #17:
BUILD SELF-WORTH

In order to see your worthiness, you have to be aware of how you're feeling and what you're saying to yourself. Your actions are based on that voice in your head, whether you want it to be that way or not. Be aware of that voice in your head that may be bringing up negativity or that limits your feelings of self-worth. Be aware of times when you are giving from a place of lack, either because you're trying to please people or because you are choosing not to focus on yourself as you focus on others.

One way that we can correct the inner voice is to use affirmations. Every morning, look at yourself in the mirror and repeat any one of the following. Choose the one that resonates the most with you, the one that addresses your inner voice.

- I'm not the nagging voice in my head.
- I deserve to treat myself like my best friend.
- I accept myself exactly the way I am.
- It's a miracle I am alive.
- I don't need to be afraid, because shit always works out.
- I can take chances and see what happens.
- I am bold.
- I can impact the world.
- I have great eyebrows, just look at 'em.
- I can manifest anything I want.

YOU GOTTA LIVE WITH INTEGRITY

Simply put, aligning what you say and do is having integrity, and it feels damn good. It gives your unconscious mind permission to respect yourself. So when you say, *I'm going to wake up early tomorrow morning and get to the gym*, and instead you wake up and hit snooze five times, you told yourself five little lies and you are outside of your integrity. When you tell your kids that you're taking them to the zoo on Saturday and then get busy painting the house, you are outside of your integrity.

When you tell yourself you are going to lose weight and then eat four doughnuts for dinner, you are outside of your integrity. When you set a goal and you procrastinate until the last minute and accomplish something half-assed, yes, you still are living outside of your integrity.

When any of these things happen, it's no surprise that you don't feel worthy. In fact, it can make you feel like shit. Let's use a mundane, easy-to-fix example that we are all guilty of from time to time (or, if you are my family, all the time). When is the last time you were late? Being late means you committed to a time and then broke the commitment. Even if *something came up,* another person's time and your integrity have taken a hit.

If you say you're going to do something, do it. If you set a time for a meeting, be there early. If your trusted doctor prescribes a treatment, try it. You are worthy of your word and commitments. Having integrity feels good.

You can't experience the positive feelings of worthiness without integrity, because you will always be judging yourself. I'm not saying that you shouldn't contribute if you don't feel worthy. Instead, start to contribute while also doing the work, including the Stimulati Experiences, to make yourself feel worthy; get as much out of making a contribution as those you are contributing to. What's more, if you contribute as promised and keep your commitments, you'll be building up your integrity.

STIMULATI LARRY ROSENFIELD: MASTERING MINDFULNESS

One of my Stimulati is Larry Rosenfield, PhD, a communications professor at the University of New Hampshire, where I went to college. He was one of my favorite professors. I took his class at the onset of my illness. He was an intense, stern man and not everyone enjoyed his class, to be polite, but I could see the kindness and caring in his face. It was clear he truly loved strengthening young minds. By the time I met him, he had retired once and returned to teaching. He had so much love for working with students.

I signed up for his class Public Speaking 101 and quickly found out Dr. Rosenfield had an alternative agenda. He had to give a class on public speaking to fit the university's curriculum, but this course turned out to be something much different. Dr. Rosenfield was a student of Buddhism, and within the context of teaching us to be better public speakers, he taught us how to be present in our lives. In the end, his class was about mindfulness.

Mindfulness is the ability to recognize what is going through your head in the present moment and then be able to let it go so that you are not always wrapped up in your thoughts about either the past or the future. It allows you to have an attitude of curiosity about your thoughts and feelings without getting attached to them. The cultivation of moment-by-moment awareness of our environment is a practice that helps us cope with the difficult thoughts and feelings that cause stress and anxiety. Rather than being led by our emotions, being influenced by negative past experiences and fears of future occurrences, or ruminating over what could be, we root the mind in the present moment and deal with life's challenges as they come up. This ability can free us from unhelpful, self-limiting thought patterns and enable us to be fully present to focus on positive emotions that increase compassion and understanding in ourselves and others.

When you're caught in crazytown in a spiral of worry, doubt, or self-defeating thoughts, mindfulness lets you recognize it so you are able to say, *These are my crazy thoughts right now. I recognize what's going on. They don't have to be my reality.* Half the battle of getting rid of negative self-talk is recognizing that it's happening. You might not be able to stop it at first, but you can teach yourself to recognize the thoughts as they appear and then link them to the reason they came up in the first place. Without that knowledge, you can't figure out why you're feeling a certain way, especially if you have a pit in your stomach or your heart is racing and you can't focus.

Dr. Rosenfield's tests and quizzes contained questions that were both random and mundane, such as *what did I say 5 minutes ago to John?* But as I came to understand his point, I realized he was teaching us to be mindful and present to exactly what was happening in the class at all times. One of the techniques he taught us was an exercise that he called getting into your comfort zone. We were instructed to close our eyes and imagine the one thing that made us the most comfortable.

I always thought about a particular sunset I would often see at Chapin Memorial Beach on Cape Cod. It is memorable because when the tide is out, the orange-and-red glow of the setting sun is reflected on the still water like a mirror, creating a double sunset experience. You can just make out the waterline on the horizon. It is so beautiful and calming that it has always stuck in my mind as a place of peace, and to this day, whenever I am on Cape Cod, I try never to miss it. This sunset became my comfort zone.

My roommate, who also took the class and sat next to me, chose the word *pants* as his comfort zone. I can still see those beat-up brown khakis now.

Dr. Rosenfield then told us to close our eyes, place our feet on the floor, and count backward from 10. We would say out loud our comfort-zone word and then the number while breathing deeply. For me, it went, *Sunset 10, sunset 9, sunset 8, sunset 7* . . . I would hear my roommate, who was quite an anxious person, counting his pants in class . . . in the shower . . . in the kitchen. This exercise was meant to settle our minds, to become relaxed enough to feel safe and comfortable in our own bodies by thinking of the thing that made us most content. In this way we could be calmer, more aware, more present, and more mindful of what was happening after the exercise was over. This little meditation training had a great impact on me. It made me think of Dr. Rosenfield as one of my most trusted mentors. When I first got ill and I was feeling poorly and my body was going numb, I went to see Dr. Rosenfield, because I trusted him and I was scared. I had to leave school to try to figure out how to get better. When I told him what was happening, he was the first person

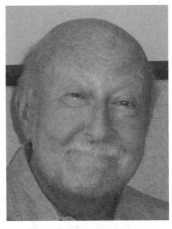

This photo shows exactly how I remember the good professor. His voicemail for his office would always end with, "You are a drop of sunshine in the dark night."

who gave me a hug and said, *Everything's going to work out okay.* He didn't know how it was going to work out; he just knew that it would. And he was right.

After I left school, I never saw him again, but I thought about him often. When I got back to school, I always looked for him, but I couldn't find him. After graduation, I searched some more. He wasn't on Facebook. He wasn't on social media. It wasn't prevalent at the time anyway.

One day I called the school, and he was no longer working there. He was lost to me.

Years later, someone from the school approached me for a donation, and I asked about Dr. Rosenfield. It turned out that he had died in 2010. The moment I heard, I had to fight back tears. I am even tearing up writing this now, 20 years after last seeing him. His kindness is still so close to my heart. I was so affected because I had never found him, or I didn't do enough to find him, and he had contributed so much to me. Then I realized that I could contribute in his honor, and I set up a scholarship in his name. When I received an incredibly touching and grateful letter from the star student who was able to continue with her studies only due to the financial support in Dr. Rosenfield's name, I felt such an incredible warmth that I cried again. And I am not a crier! His contribution had finally come full circle for me.

STIMULATI EXPERIENCE #18:
PRACTICE MINDFULNESS

This exercise is designed to enhance your ability to be nonjudgmental. The reactions we have to the sounds we are surrounded by are influenced by past experiences, but when we listen mindfully, we can achieve a neutral, present awareness that lets us hear without judgment.

Select a piece of music you have never heard before in a genre you don't typically listen to. Close your eyes and put on your headphones. Try not to judge what you think the music will sound like by its genre, title, or artist name before it has begun playing. Instead, allow yourself to get lost in the journey of sound for the duration of the song. Allow yourself to explore every aspect of the track. Even if the music isn't to your liking at first, let go of your dislike and give your awareness a chance to hear the full song without judgment. The idea is to just listen and become fully entwined with the music. If it turns out that it wasn't to your liking, you never have to listen to it again. However, it may open the door to a whole new range of pleasure.

CONTRIBUTION LEADS TO PURPOSE

You already learned that connection is the antidote to loneliness, because you can find other people with similar experiences and relate to them in a real way. That action of listening and sharing stories takes you out of yourself, out of your illness, and into a space where you can see your worthiness.

Listening to other people's stories is the easiest way into connection. Telling your story is the next level. Telling your story to make a connection is for yourself. When it comes from a place where you value yourself and have self-love and you feel worthy, contribution is the ultimate level. Telling your story with contribution is for others.

Contribution goes beyond telling the story. It is the action you take so that other people feel hope and can be inspired. And when you are contributing, you're giving something of yourself. Because you have enough, you start to build a feeling of significance that you can make an impact, as opposed to giving to please, so you don't have to focus on yourself, or because you think it's the right thing to do.

Contribution allows us to continue to progress with our health and maintain a positive state of mind. It can be as little as a gesture or as big as giving back to your community. But one of the best ways you can contribute is by sharing your story with the intention of inspiring others, not with the intention of fame. Fame or popularity can leave you feeling disconnected because you'll become more concerned with how many Likes you're getting than with how many people you're helping.

One of the ways I contribute is by volunteering at Project Sunshine in New York City. This organization is a nonprofit that provides free educational, recreational, and social programs to children and families living with medical challenges. I work with a group of teens that have lupus, and I speak with them about the challenges of going to school or getting a job when you are dealing with a chronic illness. They have many of the same concerns I did when I was their age, such as *what if I have to take a day off because I have a flare? What if I'm in the hospital for a while? Do I tell people about my illness before I take a job?*

I connect with them by sharing my own story of illness and trying to find a job. But my contribution goes beyond that story. I answer their questions, help them write their résumés, offer advice, connect them to people that may need employees, and coach them on how they should speak in an interview.

In Raina's story, featured in the last chapter, she told her story and started to connect. She set goals to become sober and clean, get a job, and reunite with her children. She accomplished those goals and gained a sense of worthiness. Then she went on to become an advocate, which is her contribution. Today she feels empowered, significant, and on the path to healing.

PURPOSE LEADS TO SIGNIFICANCE

Significance is knowing that you have a place in the world and that because of you, things can happen and change. Significance is the feeling that you mean something, that you're important, and that you have the potential to affect your surroundings. I believe that everybody has an ego-driven need to feel significant. But I do not believe that everybody inherently feels that they need to contribute. Most people are looking for significance in material ways. They buy cars. They own fancy homes or take lavish vacations. They wear their illness as a badge of honor. But neither physical objects nor martyrdom actually make us significant.

Instead, significance comes from having the awareness that you are making other lives better without a condition or control.

My career goals used to be summed up in a word: money. I can remember when I made enough money to buy my first expensive watch. It was a beautiful platinum Rolex, and it cost thousands of dollars. I would wear it with such pride, and it almost made me feel significant. If I was wearing a Rolex, it showed that I was successful and wealthy and that I must mean something. The problem was, it forced me to look at everybody else's watch and base my significance on who was wearing the more expensive watch in that moment. If it was me, I was the winner; if it wasn't, I felt defeated.

I soon learned that in New York City, there's always going to be someone with a more expensive watch. I would look at those men with envy, or I'd take it as a challenge to buy another watch. That insecurity led to my owning 10 watches, each more expensive than the next. I spent way too much time deciding which watch to wear and what events I would attend.

I once went to the Miraval resort in Arizona for a week of meditating and "releasing shame." I remember getting back from the trip and realizing that I was so much more than my watches. I was wrapping up my worth and my significance in what I owned, the material items, and I was so much more than that. I realized that feeling significant is not about the watch. I would always be measuring myself up to the next best watch or someone else's more expensive watch. Significance is more than that; it's about who you are and what you do to make a difference.

When I started studying at the Kadampa Center, my Stimulati Morten Clausen taught that if we lived on Mars and had a stack of $100 bills, those $100 bills would mean nothing. What does have meaning or true value is the way that you think and act. Everything else is an illusion. Once I understood his message, I never wore a watch again. I never had the anxiety of walking by a watch store and wondering if I could afford a particular watch or going to a party and seeing someone with a better watch and wondering if he was more successful than me. In the end, I sold 9 of the 10 watches and kept my favorite one, because of its beauty. But I don't even wear it anymore. I donated the money from selling the other watches, because they actually became more of a burden and a handcuff than the significance I craved.

Now I know that significance comes from making a contribution and helping others. Significance, worthiness, integrity, and the desire to contribute are the factors that lead to purpose. You can't have integrity, worthiness, significance, and the desire to contribute to others and still feel as though you are not enough. We are innately designed to get a euphoric feeling from helping people. Think about the adage *when you give, you receive.* Helping others makes us feel good about ourselves, which provides a real feeling of worthiness.

I am Significant

I was living in NYC, and my apartment had a beautiful terrace overlooking Gramercy Park. Every night I could see the hundreds of lights in each apartment. I'd think about all the different lives happening behind each of those windows. At first, this made me feel insignificant, because my problems couldn't possibly matter to anyone else: If I died, the world wouldn't stop.

One day I was driving to a family Christmas dinner with my niece in the car. I was looking at all the cars in the traffic on the highway and thinking the same thing, about how each car has a different life, each person has her own issues and suffering, and how we are all disconnected and insignificant.

Yet I came to the realization that because I have a deep connection to my family, I am worthy. If I died and my story was told, the people I didn't know would connect to it because of shared human experience. I realized that you don't have to be known by everyone to be significant. What's more, we are all connected. Individuality is not insignificant; it's something that actually ties us together.

STIMULATI EXPERIENCE #19:
REEXAMINE YOUR GIFTS

Living with purpose means that you are coming from a place of abundance, that you have insight into who you are, what you're passionate about, and where you can help. Get a notebook (or write in the back of this book), and go back to your gifts. Start to journal for at least 10 minutes per day. Write down how you can use your gifts to contribute. This will lead you to your purpose more quickly than you might think.

THE PSRAI RESEARCH PROVES THE IMPORTANCE OF CONTRIBUTION AND PURPOSE

At Remedy Health, we found that chronically ill people who start to contribute effectively change their story. The most likely sequence of events went something like this. People came to the website looking for hope and found what they were looking for with the Live Bold Live Now documentaries. We know they were effective because viewers started to comment on the documentaries and then began to share their own stories on the website and let other people learn from their experiences.

We studied the people who shared their stories. We found that hearing people's stories and interacting with people like you who have triumphed leads to better health outcomes. Beyond that, the people who have triumphed and who have told their stories develop an enhanced sense of well-being. They tend to stay healthy because they feel a sense of contribution. What's more, they feel an obligation to live up to being the role model. They feel a responsibility to others to keep up their end of the bargain, to keep up their health.

Keep in mind that contribution is work. It takes practice and some learning in order to feel its full benefit. However, it can create fast transformations. Once you start to feel the excitement of your significance, you will want to contribute even more. And whenever you start to have doubts, you can remember how great it feels to help someone, and you'll stop thinking about yourself. This may seem counterintuitive, but the goal is to stop thinking of yourself in a way that is unhealthy. You're there. You love yourself. You're worthy. You deserve it. Stop dwelling on the fact that you're ill and try to help someone else who may be suffering—see how that feels.

AARON LIVES WITH HIV
AND CONTRIBUTES EVERY DAY

Aaron Laxton is a program coordinator with a veteran's housing agency in St. Louis. He loves his job because he completely relates to the men and women who come to him for help. As a veteran himself, he takes great pride in improving the lives of veterans. The people he serves are homeless veterans, and he understands the poor choices they make, because he was one of them. His poor choices led to drug addiction and HIV infection.

Aaron came from a family deeply affected by drugs and mental illness. He was moved from one foster home to another, sometimes without notice or in the middle of the night. He was sexually and physically abused in foster care and struggled with depression, anxiety, and post-traumatic stress disorder. After aging out of foster care at 18, Aaron enlisted in the army. He served in South Korea, obtaining the rank of an E5 sergeant. However, in 2000, unable to keep his real identity a secret, he came out as gay to army officials. He was honorably discharged under the military's *don't ask, don't tell* policy at the time. Once again, his life was taken away from him.

Aaron says that he was kind of a train wreck when he was discharged from the military. His skills weren't valued in civilian life, and it was difficult, if not impossible, to find a job. He started using drugs to self-medicate his PTSD. As he got deeper into the cycle of addiction, he couldn't admit that he had a drug problem, even as it was making him sick. He felt it was just one more thing that made him feel inferior to others.

In 2011, Aaron was diagnosed with HIV. The first thing he did was create a video of himself coming from the doctor's office. He intuitively knew that if he connected with people and shared his story, he somehow would feel better. He posted that video on thebody.com and then made a decision to create a short video of his experience dealing with AIDS every day. His video diary is called *My HIV Journey*.

The news was so devastating that he lost the will to face the world. The first week he spent days in bed. He refused to participate in life. But by day 4, he realized he had a purpose. He started spending a lot of time consoling those closest to him.

Slowly, people started responding to his video blog, sharing comments such as *you are not alone*. Aaron felt empowered. Putting his story out in such a public place allowed him to be in control of at least some aspect of his life. He decided early on that he would show every part of his journey, the highs and the lows. He would offer advice, support, and motivation to his community, and when he shared his shortcomings, such as a relapse after being clean and sober for a full year, he hoped that others would learn from his screw-ups. On day 125, Aaron shared that he didn't have a paying job, which at the time meant that he didn't have health care, and was on the verge of eviction. He worried that he would have to pawn the equipment needed to continue making his videos. But every day, the comments he received kept him going. He saw that he was making a difference.

Aaron also found love in the midst of his illness. Not long after he was diagnosed, he met a man named Philip, and they immediately connected. Aaron felt obligated to tell Philip that he was living with HIV, and to his relief, Philip didn't care. They don't let the illness define their relationship. However, they decided to make thoughtful choices, and Philip began taking PrEP, a medication protocol to prevent him from getting infected.

Once Aaron's health stabilized, he took his outspokenness off YouTube and became an HIV activist. In 2012 he attended the International AIDS Conference in Washington, DC, and his photograph in front of the White House went viral. That was the moment he knew he wanted to be an influencer, not a bystander. Today he blogs, writes for various publications, takes on speaking engagements, and continues to create more videos. He is open and honest about his health, which allows others to come to him with their own issues. He teaches his clients to take a positive inventory of their lives every day so that they can see where they are and where they are going.

However, Aaron realized that his contribution through activism and mentoring was not always coming from an authentic place. He was still in survival mode until 2014, when he decided to take some time off and focus on himself. He needed to get to the bottom of his addiction. He entered a 90-day recovery program and, with Philip's help, came through as a conqueror. That is not to say he never struggles, but he continues to live a purposeful life: He works with other addicts and inspires them to live stronger, bolder, and better. He continues to post his videos. And he continues to raise awareness about HIV research and make a difference.

You can check out Aaron's story here: www.thebody.com/LBLN /living-with-hiv/launch.html?ic=ms.

THOUGHT IGNITER

If contribution wasn't meant to be a way of life for everyone, then why does giving back feel so empowering?

Chapter 8

LIVING A MEANINGFUL LIFE

THOUGHT IGNITER:

*How can you make meaningful choices that provide you with
the greatest sense of purpose so that you can then share your
purpose with others?*

Having a purpose in life gives you the confidence and motivation to use your gifts and contribute. At the same time, your purpose propels you to heal. It motivates you to stay on the path of achieving your goals. When you have identified your purpose and know what you're striving for and what you're supposed to be doing, you will be able to see how each goal connects with your gifts and how achieving them can lead not only to better health but also to living boldly.

The studies I mentioned in Chapter 1 show that people who have identified a purpose in life have better health outcomes. The reason is that your purpose acts like a grounding force that keeps you calmer and more centered, especially when you are faced with new obstacles or struggle. Think of it as an anchor that protects you during a tsunami. When you use your gifts for a greater good, you feel worthy and significant. Most of all, you feel bold. That boldness is the protection you can rely on when you are confronted with obstacles or setbacks or when the struggle of everyday life intensifies. Your boldness makes it easier to keep your eye on your purpose and not get caught up in the storm, because your other worries can take a back seat. You can push worry and fear about the smaller issues aside when you focus on boldly achieving your big-picture goals. Purpose teaches you that there will always be waves and that your boat is going to rise and fall but that you will still get to your destination. Small problems will no longer seem like insurmountable obstacles, and you won't get deterred as easily.

Imagine that you are a doctor whose job is to run a hospital ward filled with sick children. Every day, you make sure that you are taking care of yourself so that you can be present to take care of these children. You get up, go to work, and exercise, even if you're feeling tired or depressed. You have to keep going because of your commitment to your purpose.

Although we need to commit ourselves to one single purpose at a time, I also believe we can have a life filled with purposeful living. For example, my purpose is to give health back to the world by sharing my story in a way that ignites inspiration, hope, and action in others. But as I write this, I'm also focused on purposeful living. I'm living my passion, and I'm affecting others positively. I just adopted a 4-month-old rescue puppy. He was malnourished and had some pesky worms. Caring for him means I've been waking up at 6:30 a.m., jumping out of bed, and getting the dog outside before he goes to the bathroom in the house! But this puppy allows me to achieve a life of love and affection and fun: He is such a joy! Right now, my purpose is to raise him to become a happy, healthy, and obedient service dog, and I've noticed that when I'm taking care of him, the other things I'm typically anxious about, including what the day's going to bring, my health, or my business, seem much smaller. I don't even think about them

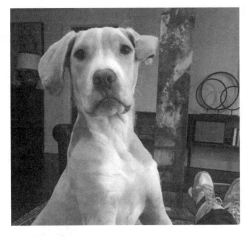

My dog, Odie. I often wonder who rescued who . . .

when I wake up now; all I think about is this puppy's well-being. That is what purpose feels like.

Now, don't get me wrong: I still have to take care of my more difficult responsibilities, and my problems don't magically disappear. They are simply smaller in perception and easier to overcome.

STIMULATI PAM WOLF: THE GIFT OF ABUNDANCE

Of all the wonderful qualities that define a life with purpose, the one that has most changed my life has been a sense of abundance. With abundance, you feel like you have everything you need, even if you're not a millionaire or in the best of health. You believe in your heart that good things are coming to you and that you will get what you need when you need it. With abundance, there is never a fear of scarcity, that feeling of *I won't have it; it's not going to happen, and there isn't enough.* Instead, the paradigm of abundance allows you to feel *I trust that it's going to work out because I am enough. When I need something, I will find it.*

When you live with a feeling of abundance, it becomes even easier to contribute, because you're not coming from a place of lacking: You have the time and energy to give to others. What's more, contribution adds to this feeling of fulfillment. Again, the more you give, the more you receive.

I learned to embrace the idea of abundance from my earliest Stimulati, my sister Pam. Pam and I did not grow up with privilege. We grew up in an urban suburb of Boston, a town called Brockton, and started both of our careers with nothing. Pam has always been a role model for me. She is 14 years older, and I watched her become a successful woman from the perspective of not only a younger brother but also a businessperson. Pam is the ultimate motivator; she had me start my first business when I was just 18, giving local kids swimming lessons at her pool. By the end of the second summer, Swim with Jim was so successful that I didn't need to work a job at college the next year (which left me more time to focus on my studies and, of course, beer and girls).

Pam's entrepreneurial spirit and can-do mindset are infectious and abundantly positive, and motivate people to move forward toward their goals. It shouldn't be a surprise that she talks a lot. She is not shy about giving out her point of view. That also comes in abundance. I had been talking about getting a puppy for 3 years. I love dogs, but I was afraid: Could I handle the responsibility? What about when I travel? Who will walk him when I am at work? Will my son love him? Pam was the one who simply said, "What are you waiting for? You love dogs; you will figure it out. Go do it and stop talking about it."

Pam and her husband of 28 years were teaching me without even knowing it: monkey see, monkey do. We model our actions around our inner circle. We use the same slang as our friends, the same catchphrases, and the same tone of voice. This is why it's important to surround yourself with people who are both positive and additive.

Pam has always had a mindset of abundance. Some people are lucky that way; this sense that she has a fullness of life now and more is coming to her is one of her gifts. She has always approached life with a combination of confidence and incredible drive.

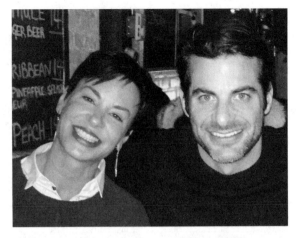

My big sis, Pam Wolf, and I at one of our many family dinners in NYC.

Because she completely trusts herself, she was able to move quickly through any fear and identify her purpose early on. She doesn't worry about lack or loss, and because of that she has gone from one success to another in both her business and personal life.

Pam started her first business when she was in college, selling hand-painted sweatshirts on her college campus in Boston. After college, she moved to New York City and started a recruiting business that was very successful. She went on to start other businesses; many succeeded, and some failed. Yet she never suffered a setback. Her failures motivated her to do something different and explore a new path.

Pam realized that her purpose was to support children to develop their emotional, physical, and artistic potential. After having two of her four children, she first started a business called the New York Kids Club and later developed the New York Preschool. They are now New York City's premier children's enrichment centers, renowned for creative and innovative classes, day camps, birthday celebrations, and special events. After the tragedy of 9/11, Pam's business model was disrupted. New

York City was in a difficult state, and young families who were her potential clients were fleeing to the suburbs. At one point the business almost went bankrupt, but she stuck with it, overcoming any fear. She had persistence, and because she knew her purpose, she believed that eventually the business would work out. Fifteen years later, as CEO, Pam oversees 300 employees, 15 locations in New York City, and even one in China. Pam is not only living in emotional abundance but also comfortably sits among the wealthiest female entrepreneurs in the United States.

Although my sister is now successful financially, she wasn't always that way. She taught me that there is no point in worrying about scarcity. Even when she wasn't financially stable or when she didn't have a family, she stayed focused on her goals. For example, my sister has always been one who says, "We can't afford to buy this piece of real estate, but we're going to buy it anyway and find a way to pay for it, because I know it's going to work out well." Today those pieces of real estate she purchased are worth millions of dollars.

She also knew that because she was living in a world of abundance, she didn't have to fear starting her family before she made money. Today she has four children and lives in New York City: That is not easy! Like anyone, Pam worries, especially about her family, but she doesn't let her worries consume her or stop her from confidently taking action in life. When her husband was diagnosed with a rare and life-threatening throat cancer, her life became absolutely daunting. Again, with the unique drive, persistence, and optimism that she applies to life, she pushed through the worry, grief, and fear, and after a long battle, together they regained his health.

More recently, Pam's world was turned upside down when she had to send her youngest son to a therapeutic boarding school in Montana, but not before he went on an extreme wilderness retreat where she did not see or talk to him for months. Dealing with her son's issues and setting up the right therapeutic programs were incredibly difficult for her: She went through extreme emotional trauma worrying about her son and making difficult choices about his care. Yet after 2 full years of trials and tribulations, her family has come out stronger than ever. I often hear her say, "You don't know pain and fear until your child is in real danger."

Back in 1998, when I first moved to New York City, I had little money and was barely hanging on to my health. I was going to happy hour at a local bar to eat the free food that came with buying a beer: not healthy but better than another package of ramen noodles. Despite all of this, I held the belief that I was going to be wealthy and healthy, because I was infected by Pam's sense of abundance. That's not to say I never grew impatient or had some fear, but I never doubted that I could have what the world had to offer. Today I have an amazing 9-year-old son and a few homes: My life is expensive. I know that money will come when I need it. That is a belief in myself that I will always have enough.

At the same time, knowing that money will come doesn't mean I don't have more goals. Someday I want to own a private jet. I have a picture of one posted on my desk. I want to be able to fly wherever I want to go, whenever I want—in style. Will I get there? Maybe, maybe not, but I'm not worried about it. I'm going to keep doing the things I'm doing that lead to a purposeful life and giving back, and I'm confident that the law of abundance will provide.

There are other people in my life who have made a lot of money, yet they're always worried they're going to lose it. Ironically, they typically do, because they don't have confidence or a feeling of abundance that even if they lose it, they'll make it again. For instance, my friend Tony is struggling with money. He hates money. He hates people with money. He has a relationship with money that is adversarial. He's told me, "I've got to make more money, but I hate it. I hate that I have to get it. I hate that it's not coming to me. I'm worked up and stressed out about money. Jim, you can't relate, because you have plenty of money. You don't know the struggles of someone without money."

I told Tony that there are millions of people who struggle without money, but there are also many people without money who are happy, living in a world of abundance, and still giving the shirt off their back to someone in need or donating to a charity. These are people who wonder how they're going to buy groceries for the week. Yet they have a feeling of abundance, and they are not obsessively worried about or hating their situation. When you hate something, you unconsciously shut your mind to it. If you are in an adversarial relationship with money, you're going to shut off your ability to make it! If Tony had gratitude for what he had and confidence that money would come, if he was open and let it, he would have a much different life and much less stress.

It is the same with your health. Live in a world of healthiness, make purposeful choices that have substance, and give back and you will achieve better health.

STIMULATI EXPERIENCE #20:
CREATE THE MINDSET OF ABUNDANCE

Developing a feeling of abundance is about creating a positive association with the things you want: health, money, family, relationships, etc. It is allowing them to become a goal without shutting down around these topics, being afraid of them, being prejudiced against them, or hating them.

Start with a realistic assessment of what you have. Let's be honest: There's a difference between *I don't have enough* and *I want more*. The latter is aspirational while the former represents scarcity. It's better to be aspirational. In fact, in order to live in abundance, you have to want more. It's not selfish to think, *I want to be super successful; I have a purpose, and I want to get paid for it; I want to have the finer things in life; I want good health, happiness, and strong relationships.*

Then the way you move from feelings of scarcity to abundance is through gratefulness. In order to change the scarcity conversation that may be your internal dialogue, focus on what you have that you are grateful for. Be grateful for the money you have, the family you are a part of, the home you live in. Be grateful that you have found your purpose or your gifts or that you have identified new goals. Maybe you have none of that? Okay, be thankful for electricity and running water, the ability to be absolutely inspired by a beautiful sunset, or the way candlelight flickers on the walls of a dark room. When you can identify what you're grateful for, you'll see that you are already living in abundance.

You can be abundant in some areas of your life and scarce in others. My abundance has always been with money: I've always been blessed with the ability to make a living. However, I've struggled with relationships. This is where I had to make a change. I had to put aside my fear and feelings of unworthiness and let love in.

Next, align your abundance with your goals. Go back to your road map. What further actions do you need to take to move yourself toward those goals? Add these new action steps to your letter. I wanted to see what parts of my life were not aligning with my purpose. I went back to the self-evaluations I've included in Chapter 1, and I realized relationships were a weakness for me, despite my clear gift of making others comfortable. Why was that? It wasn't because I hated people. When I dug deeper, I had a fear of unworthiness, and I was living in a scarce place of feeling like I didn't have enough, so I didn't connect with people. This idea of scarcity in my relationships was something that I could work on.

I created a new story of abundance. My old story about lacking relationships went like this:

The irony of living in New York is that there are so many of us, yet we are all lonely because we never talk to anyone. I avoid my doorman because small talk drives me nuts. I see the doorman, and I have to say, "Hey, Bill. How is the weather?" Then I have to walk by him five times, and every time I go out it's the same thing. I don't know my neighbors, because even though we live on top of one another, literally, we need to have a little personal space. We live one small wall apart. So for privacy, we don't make eye contact. We don't talk in the elevator. Same thing with people on the subway.

I wish I had a better relationship with my son, but he lives with his mother most of the time, and he's pissed at me. My sister is a pain in the ass, because she's so high intensity, and I can't keep a girlfriend because I get bored. I literally date a new girl every quarter.

When I think about my story when I was in survival mode, I realize now that even then I didn't believe it. As a child and in my early teens I was pure love and wanted to know and interact with everyone. When I turned that love off, out of fear and a sense of needing to protect myself, I felt wrong. Once I realized that my purpose is to affect and help people, I had to connect with others again so that I could figure out what they needed and become a positive part of their stories. So I took action: I made it a point to authentically pay attention when face-to-face with people, to listen and initiate conversations. I joined interest groups, I asked deeper questions of my doorman and cabdrivers, and I got a puppy! Now I am literally stopped by people on the street 15 times every time I walk the dog. Everybody wants to stop and pet the dog, ask me about the dog, and talk to me about the dog, and I am genuinely excited to speak with them. This is when I feel at my best.

Now I have more people in my life than ever before. I know and love my neighbors, and guess what? Once I knew them, I realized that they're not too close: It's like living with extended family. My son just has to go 5 feet down the hall to play with the children next door. My neighbors were helpful when I got locked out of my building! I am so grateful and lucky that I have these people in my life, because it makes life not only more fulfilling but also easier: Ever hear the phrase *It takes a village?* Life is hard, but when you have relationships, large and small, it makes it so much more full and abundant.

THE ULTIMATE PURPOSE: BE A STIMULATI TO OTHERS

Once I embraced abundant thinking, I was able to become my own Stimulati. I realized I intuitively had the answers that would allow me to heal. Each good decision opens the door for me to make more good decisions, especially about my health. As I healed with a feeling of abundance, I realized a calling to give to others. I recognize my purpose, and I know that I can make an impact.

The last step to living with purpose and sharing your story allows you to be a Stimulati to someone else. This contribution allows for greater abundance through connection.

"VERONICA'S" STORY: FINDING HER POWER

I met an inspiring woman in 2016. She suffers from chronic Lyme disease and came to me for guidance. I don't pretend to be a therapist but was happy to fill the role of her Stimulati and be a coach. She was excited to share her story with me but told me that I could use it in my book under one condition: I had to change her name to Veronica.

That request was a giant red flag. Why didn't this woman want me to use her real name? What part of her illness did she want to hide? Here's her story, in her own words.

In 2007, I was 42 and a working mom, and I had a full plate of the stress we all feel. But somehow I knew that was I was feeling was different from what my friends were complaining about. I was dragging around all the time. I was having numbness and tingling and shortness of breath. I had also lost a lot of weight—30 pounds—which was confusing, because nothing had changed about my diet or amount of exercise. I went to a free health screening at my office; they took my blood pressure, and it was so high that they wanted to send me immediately to the ER. I decided I'd rather see my regular doctor. When I got there I was diagnosed with a B_{12} deficiency, and I learned that one of the symptoms was anxiety. I had a stressful job at the time, and with a husband and two small children at home, I decided that in order to reduce the stress in my life I would quit working. The symptoms seemed to resolve with B_{12} shots. No more tingling, and I started to gain weight.

Around 2009, I was having major problems with my marriage. My husband suffers from depression, and he was in a funk: He hated our Alabama town and his job. I wanted us to go to marriage counseling, but he refused and chose psychotherapy instead. At that point I realized I needed my own therapist, because he would come back from his therapist angry and made it clear to me that he believed I was the cause of his problems. Our relationship was deteriorating, and it was breaking my heart. One night after a heated argument I woke up crying hysterically and, to my shock, was covered with a rash. My doctor told me it was shingles, which is caused by a compromised immune system and typically happens to much older people.

A year later, we picked up and moved to Texas, which was far away from both of our families. I didn't want to move, but I wanted to keep our family together and I thought a new setting might lift his depression. He seemed to settle down, and we were getting along better. After I had major knee surgery, my new doctor diagnosed me with a vitamin D deficiency but wouldn't continue my B$_{12}$ shots, because my levels were fine. The problem was, my levels were fine because I had been taking the shots for so long! I started to supplement on my own, yet some of my old symptoms were returning, and deep inside I knew something was wrong again. I began to feel worse than ever. I became more anxious, and I self-medicated with alcohol to try to escape my thoughts.

Here's the big problem: From the outside, my life looked fine, but I was struggling to make sense of all of these crazy symptoms that would appear and disappear just as quickly. I had neuropathy: My face would go numb. I couldn't swallow. I had no stamina for exercise. I couldn't take the heat, even though I grew up in Miami. My body temperature registered at 95 all the time, and I had constant chills and hot flashes. I couldn't remember faces and names, and my spelling was always off. I was allergic to everything I ate and was constantly covered in hives. I started having night seizures, and I ended up in the ER, where a neurologist tested me for everything under the sun and told me I was perfectly fine and that I would die of old age. He gave me antianxiety meds and Gabapentin and sent me home.

Even my dad, who was a doctor and believed that anything was worth a try, and my mother, who was a nurse, sided with the medical world. They saw the lab reports, which kept coming back as negative. They thought I was suffering from a bad marriage and anxiety, and they took me on vacation. While I was gone I felt better than I had in years, and I even began to think that I might be crazy.

As the months went by I got progressively worse, especially when I had my period. I started Googling all of my symptoms in the middle of the night. I ended up on a menopause website and found the name of a famous endocrinologist. A visit to her revealed that my B_{12} deficiency was back, my hormones were completely out of whack, and my chronic nasal allergies were connected to a gluten intolerance. She gave me methyl B_{12} shots and put me on hormones, and I changed my diet. While some of my symptoms resolved, others continued to get worse. My anxiety was through the roof, because I still believed that I hadn't gotten to the root of my problem.

When I went back to my internist, she proclaimed I had a severe anxiety disorder and gave me antipsychotic drugs. I remember leaving her office holding the prescription in my hand, asking myself, *How did I get to this place?* I was so distraught that I considered driving into oncoming traffic. Really. I never took the meds, because I knew in my heart that I wasn't crazy. And speaking of my heart, out of the blue I developed palpitations and an irregular EKG, but a full work-up at the cardiologist revealed nothing. I was constantly thirsty. My internist thought I was dehydrated and gave me a magnesium IV. My muscles started contracting and twitching, which freaked my doctor out. She didn't know what was wrong and gave me a Xanax. She ran more tests, and each confirmed my superb health. She called my husband and told him that I had a psychosomatic disorder (i.e., *your wife is crazy*). And he believed her. Who wouldn't?

I got sicker and sicker, and I was so worn down from trying to find the answers that some days I was unable to get out of bed. I went to see the head of neurology at a renowned hospital, and he told me I had fibromyalgia that he believed was psychosomatic in nature and suggested a therapist. He also gave me tramadol, a narcotic painkiller, in case he was wrong. I did not take that either, but I started to believe what the doctor was saying, that it was all in my head.

In the summer of 2015, I hosted a college reunion on Martha's Vineyard, an island off the coast of Massachusetts, where we had been going on family vacations for the past 30 years. I was sharing my story, my litany of complaints, when my college roommate looked at me and told me that my symptoms sounded like Lyme disease, which was epidemic on the island. I told her that I had already been tested for Lyme five times, but the test results always came back negative. Then she told me it didn't matter; according to the book she had been working on, Lyme is a clinical diagnosis based on a wide range of symptoms. I thought it was ironic that the book was called *Why Can't I Get Better?* The website connected to the book had a self-test, and I pulled out my phone and did it right then. We were shocked at the results: I had a score of 104, and you only needed a score of 46 to confirm a probable case of Lyme. That book, and my best friend, saved my life. I finally had some hope that I could believe my own experience and that what the doctors were telling me did not match what I knew in my heart. For the first time, I felt relieved, because I wasn't crazy.

When I got back to Texas, I booked an appointment with a Lyme-literate physician in another town, far away. He couldn't see me for 3 months, and during that time, I found out that my husband had been telling everyone in his family that I was mentally ill. I felt betrayed, alone, and scared. I found some refuge in an online Lyme forum while I waited to see the doctor. Reading the stories of other people with similar experiences gave me hope.

After carefully hearing my story and symptoms and screening me with specialized blood work, the Lyme doctor concurred that I had Lyme, Babesia, Bartonella, mold toxins, anaplasmosis, systemic candida, Bacillus, aspergillus, Mucor, Trichophyton, and mycotoxin, and toxic metals. I also had elevated levels of lead. By then I was a 50-year-old woman, affluent, white. I wasn't eating paint chips. How did I get lead poisoning?

We started treating one infection at a time. I learned about the concept of the body burden: These infections were affecting my ability to process environmental toxins. As I killed off the infection, more toxins were released, which is why it's a slowgoing process. Over the course of the first year, many of the crazy symptoms started to disappear, and for the first time I was able to think that I would someday recover. Now I am about 90 percent better.

About 8 months ago, I was listening to a podcast by Richard Horowitz, MD, the author of the Lyme book. He said that the last 10 percent of healing is an emotional and spiritual shift, and until you address that, you will not fully recover. I started going to a meditation group. I dove into the teachings and began to uncover my unconscious belief patterns. I now understand that the psyche is a real component of healing. I've had some success getting rid of the thoughts that align with fear and anger and redirecting my life to joy and serenity. I know that I'm a work in progress, but I have a deep understanding of myself now. I have days when I feel fantastic, days that are horrible, and lots of days when I wonder if I'll ever be normal again. My husband, like a lot people in the medical community, still doesn't believe in chronic Lyme. Luckily, our therapist does, and as she cautions him to keep an open mind, he's coming around. When I am having a bad day, gratitude for my life and each moment goes a long way.

At first this woman's story confused me. Some of it was inspirational and courageous. In fact, she was a powerhouse: She knew that she didn't have to take no for an answer, and she pressed on until she got the treatment that she not only needed but also deserved. At the same time her story exposed a lot of vulnerability. There were a few tells, as in poker, that expressed the secret of how she's feeling beyond the Lyme.

First, I noticed she felt her suffering and couldn't get past it. This was clear to me because within her story she made herself the victim: *no one believed me, and then my husband had his depression, and I had to take care of him. My father, who's a doctor, told me I was crazy, and he must know, because he's a doctor.*

I reminded her that we are all carrying victim stories. There is no judgment with this fact, but do victims achieve everything they want? Do they live in abundance? No, not really.

The fact that she wanted to change her name to Veronica was a clue. It showed me that she did not feel worthy inside of her story. I reminded her that she had already been telling everybody this story, including her husband, her father, her doctor, her friends, and I asked her why at this point she wanted to distance herself from it. Was it because she was not feeling worthy or because she didn't want anybody to know she had troubles with her husband? I pointed out that she was not the only person to have issues with a spouse, and she wasn't the only woman to be called crazy because she was dealing with a hard-to-diagnose condition.

Then I told her that I could help her get over the hump of the last 10 percent if she was willing to work on addressing the honest truth behind her fears. We talked about her need to please, her relationships with her husband and her family, and her perceptions about her illness. I walked her through the lessons in this book, and I told her that from reading her story, I could see that she was already incorporating many of them into her life. She was already meditating and working on self-love. She was already open to hearing other people's stories. She knew why she was sick. She was grateful for what she had. Our job was to focus on crafting her a new story and figuring out her purpose beyond her goals of healing and getting back to normal.

I asked her to imagine for an instant that she wasn't crazy, that she could help people, that her husband was going to love her because she was wonderful no matter what, and that it was okay to tell your health story. I explained that she was not defaming anyone and that she was worthy to tell her story, because she could help other people, and she should feel worthy and significant of the recognition for that. We worked together to reframe her story. I asked her to tell it differently: *I had an illness. I wasn't at my best. There's no one who can tell me that I can't get better, because I can manifest anything I want. It's not easy, and*

I'm going to take a step-by-step approach, but I'm going to fucking do it. I'm not Veronica. This is my story, truly.

In this version, her story expressed her true power, and instead of being steeped in victimhood, it was steeped in her abundance. I explained that her story is going to continue to evolve and that one of the fastest ways to induce change is to choose something specifically to be hopeful for. We tried the What Do You Want Stimulati Experience in Chapter 5, and after a few attempts, she began to see her life a little more clearly. In fact, she knew exactly what she wanted: She wanted to be taken seriously by her family. And she knew how to get it: by building her self-worth through the other exercises in this book.

My last ask was to see if she was living a purposeful life and contributing to others. I wasn't surprised at all to find that she was already mentoring several people on her favorite Lyme website. If you ask me, she is more than 90 percent healed. She is doing the work to become stronger, better, and bolder. She's writing her own book about treating her Lyme disease. And when I showed her the final version of her story for this book, she said, "You know what, Jim—you can call me by my true name, Lillian."

THOUGHT IGNITER

If you don't go after what you want,
how will you ever get it?

CHAPTER 9

PUSHING FEAR ASIDE AND BOLDLY TAKING ACTION

THOUGHT IGNITER:

Life is about moving forward and backward.
Sometimes you move forward two feet, then back one inch.
Sometimes it feels like you've moved back a foot.
The key is to try to keep moving forward, no matter what.

You've reached the finish line, and you now have the skills to live stronger, better, and bolder. Hopefully you've read through the book, been inspired by the stories, and had some aha moments that connected with your current situation. It's time to apply those skills. In your mind, you may have already started thinking about your past in a new way; you might have begun to create a new story. Along the way, you may have begun to identify your goals, and it's likely that you know your purpose. You may be thinking about connecting, or reconnecting, and figuring out ways for you to share your new story and hear some from others. These lessons in and of themselves are part of your action plan. So if you've done any or all of them, take a deep breath and congratulate yourself. You've taken that important first step without even knowing it. Now it's time to launch you toward success.

If you're still waiting for change to come to you, I'm sorry to say it isn't going to happen. If you are waiting for change, you may still feel like a victim of your circumstance. Go back and review the lessons in this book and think more deeply about how deserving you are, how much love there is for you in this world, and how worthy and grateful you can feel.

I know that the first steps toward change can be scary, and it's much easier to say, *I'll start tomorrow.* Believe me, everyone in survival mode feels this way. For example, many people with weight issues gain more weight right before they go on a diet, because they say that they're going on a diet tomorrow, so they can splurge today. Yet tomorrow never comes.

It's human nature to plan for tomorrow: *Tomorrow I'll eat better. Tomorrow I'm going to quit drinking. Tomorrow I'm going to go online and find a new therapy or a new doctor.* But planning for change and taking action are two completely different experiences. The people who plan for tomorrow yet do nothing today are actually getting worse every day, because when you're pushing something off, it means that you can have one last binge or one last splurge every day. You end up getting worse. You're progressing, but in a negative way.

Change is daunting, and as you put together the lessons in the book all at once, you may feel overwhelmed. Try to put your fear aside. What's important is not to do everything at once but to be bold enough to take that first action step. Wake up and meditate for 15 minutes before you get your day going. Say the affirmations in the shower.

Do something that will move you forward every day, and don't give up on it. Even if it's just 10 minutes, that's more time than you may have spent on yourself in quite a while. Remind yourself that you are worthy of taking care of yourself, and do it. If you're persistent, if you don't give up and you're bold and take an action step, you will see a result. It may be feeling calmer for 5 minutes or simply having a better understanding and more awareness around why you're feeling the way you are. Those results will carry you on to the next result. Opening that door will reveal more doors.

These lessons flow in a specific order, but the important part is to be bold enough to start them now. Use this book as a working manual. A great place to begin is assessing where you are now, so go back to Chapter 1 and take the evaluations if you haven't already (and if you have, go back and take them again, especially the PIL). Don't push those tests off. Sit down, take the hour, and analyze where you are now. Then review each chapter and choose one action step that you're going to take based on the Thought Igniters. Review your road map and do the first action step on your list. Today.

What motivates me to take a step forward every day is my desire to be better, to grow, and to help people. What keeps me going is when I see and feel my mood change, when I have a greater sense of calm and confidence, and when I feel better. Then I'm motivated to keep going and to take more steps. But at the beginning, I didn't take a single step forward until I had had enough of the constant struggle. I realized that I didn't have to have the pain or I didn't have to be as anxious. It was an internal drive, and it took a lot of sheer willpower.

The motivation for others might come from something outside themselves. You may want to be a better parent to your children. Perhaps you want to get to a level of health where you can be active with them physically, or you want to get to a level of mental health where you are calm enough to have more patience with them. While children become your motivator, it's still up to you to make the decision to be bold and take those first steps.

TOKEN WASN'T A RISING STAR UNTIL HE TOOK ACTION AND THEN NEVER STOPPED

Regardless of your initial motivation, your first action steps will continue to motivate you to take more actions. The boy who best embodies this chain reaction is Token. At just 17, Token has overcome an incredible number of both physical and mental challenges to become one of the most promising young rappers of his generation.

As far back as the first grade, Token realized that he was not the most upbeat kid. He told me,

> I always characterized myself as overthinking. I overthought everything, focusing on the negative, even when I was young. I thought I was really mature, and I was mature in many ways, but in other ways, not so much. Even back then, I realized that I was always angry and sad. I hated school. I hated the people I was around. I was not communicative with anybody. My house was a stressful place. At the time, I didn't know it, but now I realize that everyone in my family suffers with depression and anxiety, including me.

In elementary school, Token was pulled out of his classroom periodically for specialized language tutoring. He had a learning disability that affected his ability to process language and comprehend words. Even though he was a good student, he constant struggled in the classroom. By the time he was 10, he was formally diagnosed with a language processing disorder, depression, and an anxiety disorder.

One of the ways he dealt with his emotions was by using food as an escape. He would eat constantly, and he was an overweight child. He knew that he was eating his feelings, but he couldn't stop. He wasn't into being fit, but in the back of his mind he always remembered that in kindergarten he had been the fastest runner in the class and was conflicted with feelings of both pride and frustration surrounding that.

When he went for his annual checkup during fourth grade, he weighed 140 pounds and hated the way he looked. His father has diabetes, and because of that, his doctor told him that while he didn't have diabetes yet, he was already on the road to it. Token understood what that meant, because he watched his father take insulin shots. He hated watching his father stab himself with a needle; it creeped him out.

Token told me,

> When I learned that I could have diabetes, it disgusted me. I remember seeing a picture of a trim Randy Jackson in the doctor's office. At the time he was one of the judges on *American Idol*, and he had been overweight and then lost a bunch of weight. I turned to my mom, pointed at the picture, and said, "Can I do that? Is that possible?" She said, "Yeah, with a diet and working out, anything is possible." Something clicked in my mind right then, and I decided that I was going to lose the weight. The only way I can describe it is like a light switch. It wasn't a gradual thing. I made a decision that I was going to lose the weight forever.

Token told his mom that he wasn't going to eat anything that was unhealthy, and she fully supported him. He was already going to an after-school program at his local YMCA, and because he was a big kid and looked a little bit older, he was able to sneak into the gym every day and run for at least an hour. It became part of his routine, and over the next year, he lost 50 pounds. When he looked at himself in the mirror, he not only liked what he saw but also realized that if he put his mind to something, envisioned the end goal, and made a plan to get there, anything was possible.

That passion and understanding would stay with him no matter what he tried to accomplish. In first grade, he had written poetry, and as he was losing weight in fourth grade, he started recording it in the form of raps. The music was more therapeutic than anything else. He never had any intention of putting it out, but in fifth grade a close friend heard his mixes and was impressed.

Token told me,

> After I lost all that weight, I realized that I could transfer this same dedication into my music. I would go to school every day, and I would come right home, get my homework done, and work on my music until dinner. It was something I did constantly: constantly writing, constantly recording. I treated it like a job. That's what took me to where I'm at now. I've stayed with that mentality. It's defined who I am and how my life is going.
>
> Some people might see it as an obsession, but my single-minded focus has actually helped me a lot. It gives me more pride in myself. Specifically, when I was working out all the time, it naturally improved my mood. A lot of what I was feeling when I was younger was hatred directed toward myself. I had anger issues, and I was constantly having temper tantrums. I felt like I didn't fit in. I directed that pain back on myself, thinking, *Why am I so different?* Honestly, after throwing a temper tantrum, I would regret it so much. I would have a fight with my sister, freak out in my house, break something, or throw something. I would be so ashamed of myself, because I

was like, *why the hell did I do that?* It was a problem I had. I would lose control, and my anger would take over. But when I'm dedicated to something, whether it's losing weight or making music, I am the one in control. I am my destiny. I am the one who is going to decide my fate. Knowing that gave me a lot more pride in the power that I have by myself.

You could imagine how impressed I was when Token told me his story, as it so closely mirrors the lessons I've learned myself. Then we talked about his music, and I explained to him that his ability to tell his story not only helps him feel stronger but also can help others. He told me that his music reflects all different aspects of his life, but his story is always a part of it. He said,

> Especially the stuff I've released in the past, it represents me feeling invincible. It's like nothing can harm me, nothing can touch me. That pride has come from me putting in the work for myself and knowing my worth. I'm big on self-worth, loving yourself, and not seeking love from others in order to get your own satisfaction. My rapping represents being in control. What's in your control is how you feel about yourself. If you want to change yourself, you can do that on your own.
>
> These feelings are sometimes a topic within my music, but it's bigger than a song. It's who I am, and it's what Token represents. Even the meaning of the name Token relates to the idea of what makes you different, makes you unique. Token means *the only,* like if I was the token Jew in a Christian neighborhood or the token white kid at a black school. Token also means something of value, a gift, like a token of gratitude or a token of

appreciation. My originality wasn't my downfall. It turned out to actually be my gift. That's the idea of Token. It's something that represents me as a whole.

Seeing someone accomplish so much at just 17 inspires others, from teens to adults. Token's story shows, as his mother told him years ago, that anything is possible. No one would assume that a 17-year-old kid would have garnered millions of views on the Internet, have a genuine friendship with celebrities such as Mark Wahlberg, or have as much raw talent as he does, but his success is real.

That doesn't mean that everything comes easily to him now. He still struggles with depression sometimes, but on the whole, he says that he's happy. His purpose keeps him focused. He told me, "What keeps me focused is my hard work and putting in the time that I do. Like we were saying before, that's where I found my worth. That's what defines me as a person over what the depression would ordinarily do. I can overcome that through my feelings of self-worth."

By this point in the interview I was literally holding my hand to my mouth. I explained to Token that people who have a strong purpose in life, who see how they fit into the world and the big picture, have better health. Just knowing how you fit in, what your place is, and what your goals are improves your health outcome. He was surprised to hear it, but at the same time he said it made sense to him. "I totally get it," he told me. "I found my purpose early, and that has helped me so much."

Token's success in accomplishing his first goal of losing weight led him to believe that he could accomplish his goal of writing music and rapping. Once you start to see the results and achieve, you will gain greater confidence and motivation to achieve the next goal on your list. You can learn more about Token's journey at www.facebook.com /UPROXX/videos/10154319275451337/.

DON'T LET SETBACKS DETER YOU

Without a doubt, moving forward means that every once in a while, you're going to stumble. In fact, I stumble all the time, and not because I walk with a limp. I still find myself caught in the trap of thinking, *I'm not good enough*. I'll start thinking about old love relationships and wonder what I did wrong. When I'm about to give a speech in front of a large group for the first time, I worry, *do I have anything to teach these people?*

A setback could be a death in the family, a relapse in your illness, or just a bad day. But when negative thoughts and feelings come on, you have to correct yourself. Sometimes the corrections are a simple change of body movement, and you can push them out of your mind quickly. Sometimes you can lean on an affirmation. *I'm calm, I'm confident, and everything always works out for me* is the affirmation that does wonders for me. Sometimes it's as easy as saying to yourself, *You can do this* or *You're worth it*.

But most importantly, when you are faced with a setback, you need to put your fear aside and reaffirm your goals. Dig deep into your will-power, your persistence, and your resilience. It may take a little bit longer than you would like to climb out of it and back into a place of well-being. Forgive yourself for that and allow yourself to feel the way you're feeling. See if you can have some awareness around why you stumbled. You don't have to stop those feelings immediately, but I can guarantee that once you are aware of where they are coming from, it's much easier to move on. Then ask yourself, *what can I do to get out of this negative place?*

The answer is your purpose. Think about Aaron's story in Chapter 7. When you relapse like Aaron did or when something bad happens, you don't have to start at the beginning. Perhaps you take a single step back and do what calls you the most. Aaron had a relapse, and he went back to what he did the first day when he found out that he was HIV positive: He spoke about it publicly. He did a video blog and came back.

When I'm feeling bad or I have a relapse, I often reach out to friends and family to try to connect. I try to be motivational to myself, reminding myself that I'm calm, confident, and everything works out for me in some way or another. Then I focus on my purpose, and before long, I'm back.

I'm also a believer that everything happens for a reason, and that includes setbacks. Recently I was doing everything right and feeling great. I was going to the gym 5 days per week, meditating often, and ticking off my accomplishments that were connected to my road map. And just when everything was going right, I broke a toe. For some people, that's not a big deal. But when you walk with a limp to begin with and you have only one good, strong leg and you break a toe, it makes it almost impossible to walk. Worst of all, it was my big toe, and it's what I base all of my balance, power, and walking on.

I could walk, but I was slow, hobbled, and in a lot of pain. I still had to travel through airports and do things. My mindset went spiraling into a variety of *poor me* scenarios. I started worrying, *my body's so screwed up, even this small problem is a disaster. What happens if something big happens? What if I broke a hip? What's going to happen when I'm 80?* I started to feel sick, and I started to limit myself. I stopped going to the gym because of the pain, and it threw off my entire routine. I became depressed, and I stopped pushing myself to be social. I was invited to a wedding, and I chose not to go. I said to myself, *I'm not going to be able to make it.* I was supposed to go on a white-water rafting trip and to another event for a good friend, and I canceled both, because I lost confidence in myself physically.

Even as the toe healed and I started to walk better, with less pain, I was stuck in the routine of *I can't.* I didn't snap out of it until I forced myself to do more physical activity despite the pain and forgave myself for not being able to do what I wanted and what I expected my body to do. Then I could see that in time my toe would heal, and although there'd be some pain, I could still walk differently and get through. I stuck with my mantra *everything always works out for me*, and as my toe began to heal, I began to feel better. I made a conscious decision to be bold and to go back to *Oh, what the fuck, do whatever it takes*, and although I didn't want to go to the gym or I didn't feel like I could work out with a trainer, I did.

The trainer introduced me to a new orthopedist to monitor my toe. He told me about new treatments and therapies in orthopedics that could help me. He also fit me for a new brace for my weak leg, and that new brace helped me walk better and strengthen another part of my hip on the right side. That has led to making walking more comfortable and efficient. Then the doctor found a new anti-inflammatory medication that helped with my joint pain. We started talking about using Botox to treat some of the spasticity in my muscles so I could walk with more ease, and that led to an inquiry about stem cell research. Next I was introduced to a woman who is familiar with a stem cell therapy hospital in Panama run by American doctors that is doing cutting-edge stem cell therapy that helps heal different issues with the spinal cord. So my broken toe that put me in a spiral of depression and *woe is me* thinking actually is helping me heal.

When you're living boldly, you're taking action, because you're not allowing fear to stop you. Find the thing that's going to spark you. You need to be bold enough and not give up, and you need to trust that the work you've done already will make setbacks shorter. Some of the lessons in this book may resonate with you more than others. When you are faced with a setback or when you're in your darkest hour, try what works best for you. Remember the lesson from the book that offered the most comfort. You may need to start meditating more so that you can release anxiety, or you can try exercising more (I know that increases my endorphins). Or call someone and connect, tell them that you love them or that you need their help.

Whatever happens, know that your setbacks might be the thing that will eventually propel you forward. If that terrible thing, the broken toe, hadn't happened, then I wouldn't have moved forward five steps to having access to and knowledge of a stem cell treatment facility in Panama that is hard to get into.

The bad things in life are not always bad. They may be an obstacle, they may feel bad, and they may cause some pain or discomfort. Life might not work out the way you think it should, but it's going to lead to something. And if you stay open, resilient, and hopeful, you can make your life work out the best possible way. If you never give up, your obstacles become opportunities.

IT IS TIME TO BE, DO, HAVE: THE 21-DAY STIMULATI EXPERIENCE TO CEMENT YOUR SKILLS

It's easy to read a book, have a few aha moments, glance through the takeaways, and then walk away without making any real changes. But that's not what this book is really about. Becoming bold takes using these new skills habitually. After all, what is the use of knowing how to play the piano if you never strike a key?

New habits require following a new routine, so I created one for you for the next 21 days. The experience sets you up to win by following a schedule to practice your new skills and apply them to your new Road Map. Please do not think of this as work. You may be thinking about skipping this and coming back to it later. You may think, "I will start tomorrow," or, "I will do this on my vacation next month, or after my next treatment, or when the kids are busy with such and such," but *don't put this off!* The hardest part is taking the first initial step. Once you do, the proverbial ball will start rolling. So, please—with some resolve and some boldness—start right now.

DAY 1

Start this step immediately after you read this. The time, the place, the situation doesn't matter.

STEP ONE: Find something to write on, anything—a napkin, or the blank pages in the back of the book. Also, find something to write with, anything—your kid's crayon, your lipstick—and write these sentences:

Congratulations, [your name]! You have officially started your new life. You chose to put yourself first, to accept and stand up for yourself, and take time to heal and become stronger. I am proud of your initiative and follow-through. I am feeling so good, and it's only been a few short weeks. Thank you for taking the first bold step.

With love and respect,

Your future self

STEP TWO: Read it aloud five times before bed tonight.

You got this; congratulations.

DAY 2

STEP ONE: This is the hardest part. Set your alarm to wake up one hour earlier than usual. As you set your alarm before bed, promise yourself that even though you are going to be tired, you are not going to hit the snooze button. Not even once.

STEP TWO: Don't break your promise about the snooze button, and get up—quickly.

STEP THREE: Immediately take a hot shower to absorb those good mood-producing negative ions. Two seconds before you get out, turn the water to freezing cold, a short shock to the system.

STEP FOUR: Find a comfortable, quiet place and do Stimulati Experience #2, the Metta Bhavana, for 10 to 12 minutes.

STEP FIVE: Stretch, do a breathing exercise or light calisthenics to get your heart rate up for 7 minutes, and follow that with setting an intention that can keep you on track for the day. Complete this sentence (write it down, right here):

My intention for today is _____.

STEP SIX: Eat a healthy breakfast. (Do you skip breakfast? Not anymore.) By healthy, I mean no sugar, aspartame, high-fructose corn syrup, or simple carbs—that stuff is literally killing you and keeping you sick (just do a simple Google search to see what I mean).

STEP SEVEN: Don't forget lunch! No sugar, corn syrup, or simple carbs.

STEP EIGHT: Please snack, but do your future self a favor and skip snacks that have sugar, aspartame, or high-fructose corn syrup.

STEP NINE: Before bed, write down five things you are grateful for, and one thing you would like to let go.

I'm grateful for:

1. _____

2. _____

3. _____

4. _____

5. _____

I let go of:

_____

_____

Awesome day, congrats!

Repeat Day 2 with a few changes. Don't forget to keep your commitment to getting up and not hitting snooze! It's an immediate integrity builder.
Things to add:

1. In Step Four, add three affirmations from Stimulati Experience #17.

2. Try watching 1 less hour of television and go to bed 45 minutes earlier.

If you are limiting or cutting out sugar, you may feel a little off, but rest assured that at the end of the 21 days, you will feel better than ever. Do your best here!

Write down your intention here:

My intention for today is _____.

Write down your thoughts for Step Nine here:

I'm grateful for:

1. _____

2. _____

3. _____

4. _____

5. _____

I let go of:

_____

_____

DAY 4

Creating habits requires repetition. Today we'll strengthen our skills by repeating Day 3 with the following additions:

1. After a healthy breakfast, start creating your Road Map.

2. In Step Four, increase your meditation practice to 15 minutes.

3. In Step Five, increase your exercise and breathing to 12 minutes.

4. After Step Nine, add a rule: No social media for 1 hour before bed.

Write down your intention here:

My intention for today is _____.

Write down your thoughts for Step Nine here:

I'm grateful for:

1. _____

2. _____

3. _____

4. _____

5. _____

I let go of:

_____

_____

How are you feeling? Are you getting up and not hitting snooze, and limiting your sugars, simple carbs, corn syrup, and aspartame?

Remember, meditation is a practice, so don't get frustrated if your mind wanders. Just notice when it does and try to come back to center.

DAY 5

Repeat Day 4 with this addition:

1. Commit to finishing your Road Map. There's a fill-in version on page 221.

Write down your intention here:

My intention for today is _____.

Write down your thoughts for Step Nine here:

I'm grateful for:

1. _____

2. _____

3. _____

4. _____

5. _____

I let go of:

_____

_____

DAY 6

Repeat Day 5—healthy habits are a-formin'.
   Additions:

1. At some point before bed, do Stimulati Experience #5.

2. Choose one action to implement from your Road Map.

3. Try not engaging with social media from dinnertime to the end of the evening.

Write down your intention here:

My intention for today is _____.

Write down your thoughts for Step Nine here:

I'm grateful for:

1. _____

2. _____

3. _____

4. _____

5. _____

I let go of:

_____

_____

DAY 7

Repeat Day 6 and replace Stimulati Experience #5 with Stimulati Experience #6.

Write down your intention here:

My intention for today is _____.

Write down your thoughts for Step Nine here:

I'm grateful for:

1. _____
2. _____
3. _____
4. _____
5. _____

I let go of:

_____

_____

DAY 8

Surprise, surprise! Repeat Day 7 but replace Stimulati Experience #6 with Stimulati Experience #8 (yes, skip #7 for now).

Write down your intention here:

My intention for today is _____.

Write down your thoughts for Step Nine here:

I'm grateful for:

1. _____
2. _____

3. _____

4. _____

5. _____

I let go of:

_____

_____

Repeat Day 8. Don't forget to set your intentions for the day.

Write down your intention here:

My intention for today is _____.

Write down your thoughts for Step Nine here:

I'm grateful for:

1. _____

2. _____

3. _____

4. _____

5. _____

I let go of:

_____

_____

DAY 10

Repeat Day 9.
   Additions:

1. Do Stimulati Experience #18.

Write down your intention here:

My intention for today is _____.

Write down your thoughts for Step Nine here:

I'm grateful for:

1. _____

2. _____

3. _____

4. _____

5. _____

I let go of:

_____

_____

DAYS 11–20

For the next 10 days, repeat Day 9. You should be starting to feel more energized, have a greater sense of calm, less pain, and a greater sense of purpose.

   Every day, write down your thoughts for Step Nine, and your intention for the day.

DAY 11

My intention for today is _____.

I'm grateful for:

1. _____
2. _____
3. _____
4. _____
5. _____

I let go of:

_____

_____

DAY 12

My intention for today is _____.

I'm grateful for:

1. _____
2. _____
3. _____
4. _____
5. _____

I let go of:

_____

_____

DAY 13

My intention for today is _____.

I'm grateful for:

1. _____
2. _____
3. _____
4. _____
5. _____

I let go of:

_____

_____

DAY 14

My intention for today is _____.

I'm grateful for:

1. _____
2. _____
3. _____
4. _____
5. _____

I let go of:

_____

_____

DAY 15

My intention for today is _____.

I'm grateful for:

1. _____
2. _____
3. _____
4. _____
5. _____

I let go of:

_____

_____

DAY 16

My intention for today is _____.

I'm grateful for:

1. _____
2. _____
3. _____
4. _____
5. _____

I let go of:

_____

_____

DAY 17

My intention for today is _____.

I'm grateful for:

1. _____
2. _____
3. _____
4. _____
5. _____

I let go of:

_____

_____

DAY 18

My intention for today is _____.

I'm grateful for:

1. _____
2. _____
3. _____
4. _____
5. _____

I let go of:

_____

_____

DAY 19

My intention for today is _____.

I'm grateful for:

1. _____
2. _____
3. _____
4. _____
5. _____

I let go of:

_____

_____

DAY 20

My intention for today is _____.

I'm grateful for:

1. _____
2. _____
3. _____
4. _____
5. _____

I let go of:

_____

_____

DAY 21

Congratulations, you made it! Today is a day you should take for yourself. Give yourself permission to focus on your health without any guilt, shame, or preoccupation.

Today is a day to focus on completing Stimulati Experiences #7, 11, 13, and 20.

Start imagining what your life can now look like, starting on Day 22, and how you will start to contribute to others.

FINAL SUGGESTIONS TO HELP YOU SUCCEED

I know there's a lot to take in. These lessons aren't always easy, and the exercises might bring up emotions and issues that are difficult to process. That's why I think this book is most effective when you read it two or three times. The second time, follow these tips.

1. **TAKE NOTES.** My mother taught me never to write inside a book, but she was not right about everything! I give you permission to make a mess. Underline and highlight the ideas that spark your interest. See where the Thought Igniters take you: Write down how they've inspired you and what new action steps you can take. Write down your road map on the pages provided at the end of the book, and don't lend this to anyone (make your friends get their own copy, and thank yourself for me).

2. **FOCUS ON YOUR ROAD MAP.** This is the major takeaway, folks. It's the plan that will show you how to implement small changes in your life that lead to big results. But don't stop thinking of actions once you've written your road map. Be on the lookout for new ways to make changes. Remember, positive change begets more positive change.

3. **START TODAY.** When you read this book through again, do at least one of the experiential exercises every day. Old patterns are easier to maintain than new behaviors, which require far more effort and vulnerability. The more quickly you begin to disrupt your limiting thoughts and beliefs, the more successful you'll be at developing new patterns.

4. **BE ACCOUNTABLE TO YOURSELF.** Don't let yourself down. Make sure you're following your road map, checking in and achieving it, and going back and taking the tests again. The underlying message of this book is that you need to be there for yourself, loving yourself, feeling worthy, being accountable to yourself. It's up to you, baby!

5. **SHARE WITH OTHERS.** This book and the lessons you've learned can become a part of your new story. Nothing would bring me greater joy. Rephrasing what you've learned and then publicizing it anywhere— social media, a bathroom wall, whatever—creates a public record of your thoughts. (Plus, it's good publicity for me.) But most of all, sharing your story and speaking about your journey give others permission to start theirs. It all comes back around to purpose.

THOUGHT IGNITER

What will you now do to spark change?

RECOMMENDED READING LIST

A New Earth: Awakening Your Life's Purpose | Eckhart Tolle

Around the Year with Emmet Fox: A Book of Daily Readings | Emmet Fox

Breaking the Habit of Being Yourself: How to Lose Your Mind and Create a New One | Joe Dispenza

E-Squared: Nine Do-It-Yourself Energy Experiments That Prove Your Thoughts Create Your Reality | Pam Grout

Happier: Learn the Secrets to Daily Joy and Lasting Fulfillment | Tal Ben-Shahar

How to Raise Your Self-Esteem: The Proven Action-Oriented Approach to Greater Self-Respect and Self-Confidence | Nathaniel Branden

Living Beautifully with Uncertainty and Change | Pema Chödrön

Man's Search for Meaning | Viktor Frankel

Mind Your Body: 4 Weeks to a Leaner, Healthier Life | Joel Harper

Spontaneous Healing: How to Discover and Embrace Your Body's Natural Ability to Maintain and Heal Itself | Andrew Weil

The Gifts of Imperfection: Let Go of Who You Think You're Supposed to Be and Embrace Who You Are | Brené Brown

The Healing Dimensions: Resolving Trauma in Body, Mind, and Spirit | Brent Baum

The Tapping Solution: A Revolutionary System for Stress-Free Living | Nick Ortner

The Universe Has Your Back: Transform Fear to Faith | Gabrielle Bernstein

The Way of Silence: Engaging the Sacred in Daily Life | David Steindl-Rast and Alicia von Stamwitz

Unlimited Power: The New Science of Personal Achievement |
  Tony Robbins

You Matter: 7 Practices of Living a Life of Purpose | Melvin Miller and
  Federica Baldan

Notes

INTRODUCTION

1. Ng, M.Y. and W.S. Wong. "The Differential Effects of Gratitude and Sleep on Psychological Distress in Patients with Chronic Pain." *Journal of Health Psychology* 18, no. 2 (February 2013): 263–71. doi: 10.1177/1359105312439733.

CHAPTER 1

1. Rohleder, N. "Stimulation of Systemic Low-Grade Inflammation by Psychosocial Stress." *Psychosomatic Medicine* 76, no. 3 (2014): 181–189.

2. Fredrickson, B., et al. "A Functional Genomic Perspective on Human Well-being." *PNAS* 110, no. 33 (2013): 13,684–89.

3. Boyle, P., A. Buchman, L. Barnes, and D. Bennett. "Effect of a Purpose in Life on Risk of Incident Alzheimer Disease and Mild Cognitive Impairment in Community-Dwelling Older Persons." *Archives of General Psychiatry* 67, no. 3 (2010): 304–310.

4. Boyle, P., et al. "Effect of Purpose in Life on the Relation Between Alzheimer Disease Pathologic Changes on Cognitive Function in Advanced Age." *Archives of General Psychiatry* 69, no. 5 (2012): 499–505.

5. Koizumi, M., H. Ito, Y. Kaneko, and Y. Motohashi. "Effect of Having a Sense of Purpose in Life on the Risk of Death from Cardiovascular Diseases." *Journal of Epidemiology* 18, no. 5 (2008): 191–196.

6. "The Adverse Childhood Experiences Study: A Springboard to Hope," www.acestudy.org/index.html.

7. Bornstein, David. "Putting the Power of Self-Knowledge to Work." *New York Times*, August 23, 2016.

8. Crumbaugh, J. "Cross-Validation of Purpose in Life Test Based on Frankl's Concepts." *Journal of Individual Psychology* 24, no. 1 (1968): 74–81.

CHAPTER 2

1. Wallace, R. K. and H. Benson. "The Physiology of Meditation." *Scientific American* 226 (February 1972): 84–90.

2. Fredrickson, B., et al. "Open Hearts Build Lives: Positive Emotions, Induced through Loving-Kindness Meditation, Build Consequential Personal Resources." *Journal of Personality and Social Psychology* 95, no. 5 (2008): 1,045–62.

3. Blanchfield, A.W., et al. "Talking Yourself Out of Exhaustion: The Effects of Self-Talk on Endurance Performance." *Medicine & Science in Sports & Exercise* 46, no. 5 (2014): 998–1,007.

CHAPTER 4

1. Malone J.C., et al. "Adaptive Midlife Defense Mechanisms and Late-Life Health." *Personality and Individual Differences* 55, no. 2 (July 2013): 85–89.

CHAPTER 6

1. Burke, M. and R.E. Kraut. "The Relationship Between Facebook Use and Well-Being Depends on Communication Type and Tie Strength." *Journal of Computer-Mediated Communication* 21 (2016): 265–281. doi: 10.1111/jcc4.12162.

CHAPTER 7

1. Bogdanos, Maria. "World of Psychology: Signs of Codependence & Codependent Behavior." Psychcentral.com (blog), April 4, 2013, http://psychcentral.com/blog /archives/2013/04/04/signs-of-codependence-codependent-behavior.

My Road Map

Over the next 90 days, I will:

Mental Health

Goal: _____

_____

Action:

   1. _____

_____

   2. _____

_____

   3. _____

_____

   4. _____

_____

Physical Health

Goal: _____

_____

Action:

   1. _____

_____

   2. _____

_____

3. _____

4. _____

Relationships

Goal: _____

Action:

1. _____

2. _____

3. _____

4. _____

Contribution

Goal: _____

Action:

1. _____

2. _____

3. _____

4. _____

JOURNAL

INDEX

Boldface page references indicate photographs and illustrations. Underscored references indicate boxed text.

C

Caregivers, 150–51
Challenges, strength through overcoming, 38
Change
    in author's stories, 3–5, 121
    motivation for, 191
    moving forward every day, 190–91
    planning vs. taking action for, 190
    setbacks, 197–200
    starting today, 191, 216
    starting tomorrow, 190
    in stories, doubts signaling need for, 57
    stories changed by contribution, 163
    stories changed through suffering, 37
    waiting for, 190
    What-Ifs for, 8–9
Clausen, Kadam Morten, 37
    Andersen's example of teachings of, 40–41
    author's experience with, 35–37
    on materialism and meaning, 161–62
    truth of now as the only time taught by, 37–40
    universal truth of suffering taught by, 36
Codependency
    basing your value on, 151–52
    in caregivers, 150–51
    contribution vs., 152
    pleasing behavior leading to, 150
    signs of, 151
Color framing technique
    author's experience with, 75–76
    Baum's development of, 73–75
    Stimulati experience, 76–77
Comfort zone practice, 156–57
Concentration camp survival, 9
Connecting to others. See also Loving others; Support
    beyond self-love, 95
    fear of disconnection, 77–78
    inspiring hope by, 116–17
    with love, 101–2
    significance in, 163
    by stories, 159
    through suffering, 36–37
Conscientiousness (personality trait), 19

Contribution. See also Helping others
    abundance aiding, 172
    benefits of, 164
    codependency vs., 152
    Laxton's journey to, 164–67
    leading to purpose, 159–60
    not needed universally, 160
    significance from, 162
    stories changed by, 163
Contribution goals, 138
Conversation starters, 101–2
Core-belief story, 139–40
Cortisol, 6–7, 96
Courage, in storytelling, 78
Crohn's disease, Everest climb with, 117–19
Curiosity, mixing with resiliency, 132
Curtis, Jim, **12**
    abundance mindset of, 175
    affirmation used by, 51
    challenges as a trader, 4–5, 55–56, 83
    color framing experience of, 75–76
    dog, Odie, 170, **171**
    doubts encountered by, 56
    Ecuadorian shaman met by, 122–24
    experience with shame, 61–64
    false hope experienced by, 104–6, 110–11
    focus on hopes and dreams by, 107
    Frankl's influence on, 11
    gifts of, 128
    goals of, 133–34
    Lee's treatment of, 34–35
    life stories changed by, 3–5, 121
    lovesickness of, 81–83, 95
    new story lived by, 125–26
    Pam (sister) as role model for, 172
    as Project Sunshine volunteer, 159–60
    Purpose in Life theory's influence on, 11
    pushing emotions down by, 78
    reaffirmation of hope by, 106
    Rosenfield's reassurance of, 157
    search for significance by, 161, 162–63
    self-forgiveness by, 67–68
    self-worth doubted by, 147–48
    setbacks by, 198–99
    soul journey experience of, 112–14
    Spatafora's work with, 126–27, 128